NOW OR NEVER

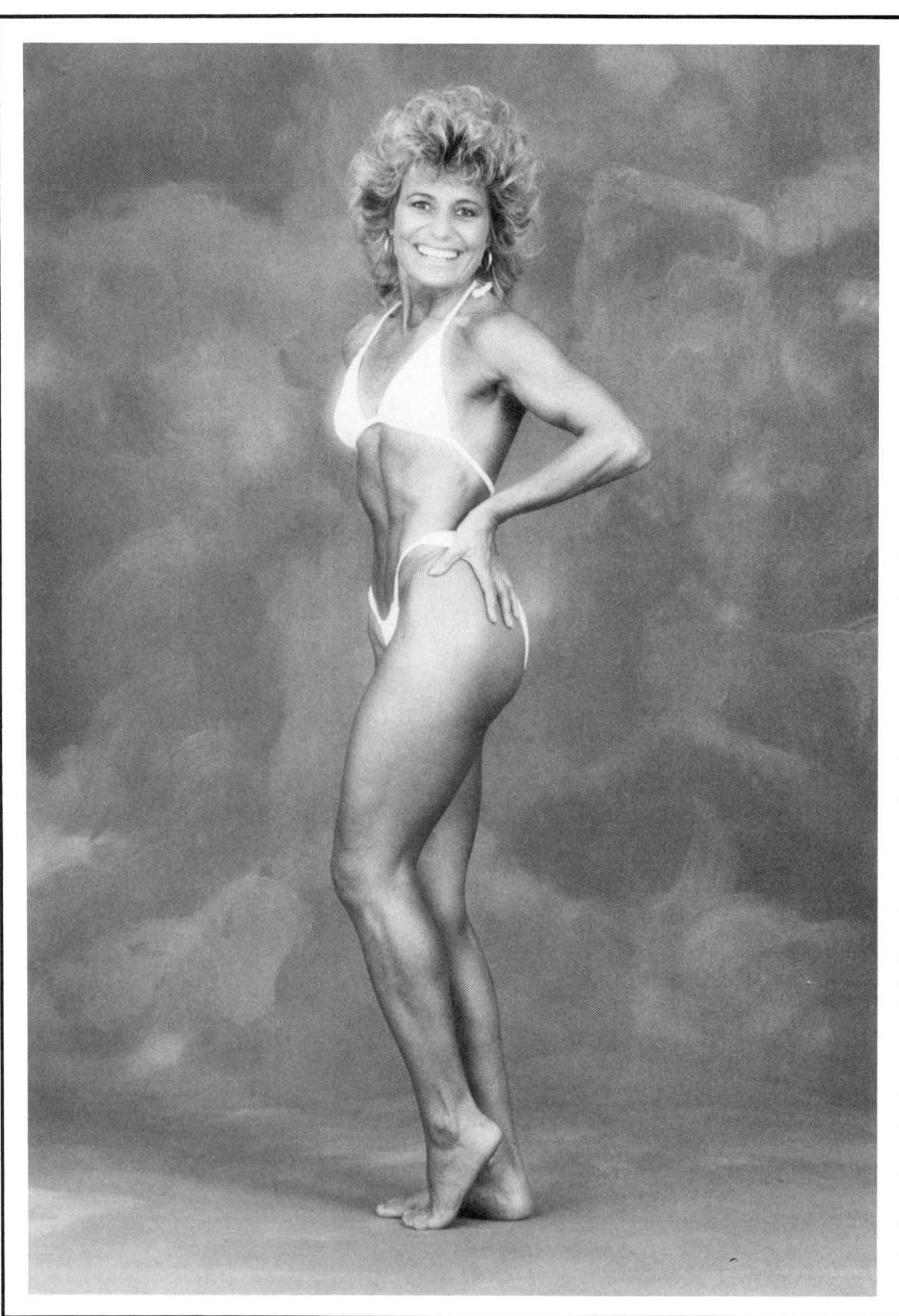

NOW OR NEVER

Keep your body young, fit and firm—
with the weight training program
that works even as you age.

Joyce Vedral, Ph.D.

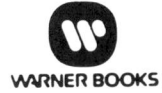

WARNER BOOKS

A Time Warner Company

If you purchase this book without a cover you should be aware that this book may have been stolen property and reported as "unsold and destroyed" to the publisher. In such case neither the author nor the publisher have received any payment for this "stripped book."

A Note from the Publisher

The ideas, procedures and suggestions contained in this book are not intended as a substitute for consulting with your physician. All matters regarding your health require medical supervision. Please consult your doctor before embarking on this or any fitness program.

Book design by Giorgetta Bell McRee

Cover design by Jackie Seow
Cover photo by Bill Charles
Black and white photos by Paul Goode
Hair and makeup by Diane Matthews
Cover leotard by Capezio
Workout leotard by Capezio
Gym shoes by Reebok
Gym backgrounds courtesy of Madison Avenue Muscle,
    New York, New York
Free weights by T. K. Star, made by T. K. Engineering,
    Mount Vernon, New York
Eagle gym machines by Cybex, Ronkonkoma, New York
Jump rope by Triangle Health and Fitness Products, Raleigh,
    North Carolina
Dress by Valentino
Suit by St. John
Polka dot jacket by Albert Nippon
Fashion coordination by Dora Franco and Lorraine Garville,
    Fifth Avenue Club, Saks Fifth Avenue, New York, New
    York

Copyright © 1986 by Joyce L. Vedral
All rights reserved.
Warner Books, Inc., 666 Fifth Avenue, New York, NY 10103

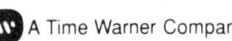 A Time Warner Company

Printed in the United States of America
First Printing: July 1986
10 9 8 7

Library of Congress Cataloging-in-Publication Data

Vedral, Joyce L.
  Now or never.

  Includes index.
  1. Physical fitness for women. 2. Weight lifting.
I. Title.
GV 482.V43 1986   613.7'045   85-31468
ISBN 0-446-37010-X (pbk.) (U.S.A.)

ATTENTION: SCHOOLS AND CORPORATIONS

Warner books are available at quantity discounts with bulk purchase for educational, business, or sales promotional use. For information, please write to: **Special Sales Department, Warner Books, 666 Fifth Avenue, New York, NY 10103.**

**ARE THERE WARNER BOOKS YOU WANT
BUT CANNOT FIND IN YOUR LOCAL STORES?**

You can get any Warner Books title in print. Simply send title and retail price, plus 50¢ per order and 50¢ per copy to cover mailing and handling costs for each book desired. New York State and California residents, add applicable sales tax. Enclose check or money order—no cash, please—to: Warner Books, PO Box 690, New York, NY 10019. Or send for our complete catalog of Warner Books.

To all the women who pick up this book and decide that it's "Now or Never." Good luck!

Acknowledgments

★ Thank you, Joe Weider, for discovering and making available the basic principles of bodybuilding through your magazines and books.

★ Thank you, Kathy McBride, for your talented editing and relentless enthusiasm.

★ Thank you, Gus "the Comrade" Stephanidis, for being my good-natured trainer and cohort.

★ Thank you, Barbara Vale, Terry Perine, Roberta Robinson, and Ellen Carter, for daring to show women how to become an "after."

★ Thank you, Jackie Merri Meyer, for your creative and sensitive art direction on the cover.

★ Thank you, Bob Oskam, for your sensitive copyediting.

★ Thank you, Karen Demilia, for your helpful advice on hairstyle and clothing.

★ Thank you, family and friends, for your unwavering belief that this book is needed *now or never.*

Contents

	Preface	xi
1.	THE TOTAL BODY LIFT	1
2.	OUT OF SHAPE? LUCKY YOU!	11
3.	WHO'S IN CONTROL—YOUR BODY OR YOUR MIND	21
4.	TIMING	37
5.	WORKOUT FUNDAMENTALS	47
6.	PREPARATION FOR BEGINNING	67
7.	THE GYM WORKOUT	85
8.	THE HOME WORKOUT	155
9.	DIET	187
10.	BOMBING PROBLEM AREAS	211
11.	BEFORE AND AFTER	217
12.	FOREVER FIT	229
	Bibliography	233
	About the Author	235
	Index	237

Preface

It is a simple matter to reverse the physical effects of aging—the atrophy of the muscles which takes place every year after the age of thirty. The method is the creation of more muscle than that which is being lost.

The program presented in this book, when followed carefully, enables one to place firm muscle under previously sagging skin. By using the empirically proven "split routine," and "pyramid" system used by champion bodybuilders and athletes, it is possible to achieve the look of a total body lift in less than a year's time, and to see impressive improvements as early as one month after beginning this program.

In addition, the creation of muscle assists in the mineralization of bone, helping to create strong healthy bone so that those who work out with this program achieve better posture and improved bone structure as they age instead of going in reverse and appearing slouched and withered. Since decalcification of bone is a problem for most women as they approach their thirties and beyond, the development of muscle can head off that problem so that it most likely will never occur.

I have been the sports medicine physician of Olympic Champions, athletes, bodybuilders, celebrities, and the general public for the past fifteen years (in Los Angeles, California). During that time, I have witnessed the transformation of the bodies of literally thousands of men and women who were willing to invest a number of hours a week in intelligent split routine weight training.

By working out with weights in the manner described in this book, women will be able not only to replace muscle being lost, but to stimulate muscle which has never previously been developed. This muscle, when formed, places itself under previously loose, sagging skin and creates a tight, toned, shapely body. Instead of becoming weaker with age, women who follow this program become stronger. Instead of feeling as if they are "falling apart" as they go into their thirties, forties, and beyond, women who follow this program feel as if they are well put together—more so than ever before. Instead of walking with a shuffle and slumping over, women on this program tend to walk with a spring in their step and an upright posture—an athletic stride.

Modern medical science has proven that it is not necessary to wither and atrophy as you get older. In fact, you can become more muscular and stronger and appear younger.

In summary, it is not "age" that makes us old, but rather disuse. This program provides the most economical method of developing and using muscle groups for every major part of the body, and women who follow it see themselves transformed into looking and feeling ten years younger in less than a year.

Walter F. Jekot, M.D.
Los Angeles, California

Dr. Jekot is an internationally known sports medicine physician who practices in Los Angeles, California. He is a member of the American College of Sports Medicine and is also a National Physique Judge for men and women. Dr. Jekot is the editor of his own monthly fitness newsletter, *Healthstyles USA*. He has recently completed working with Lou Ferrigno and his wife, Carla, on their video, "Body Perfection."

He judges the biggest contests in the world: Mr. Olympia, Miss Olympia, and the World Championships.

NOW OR NEVER

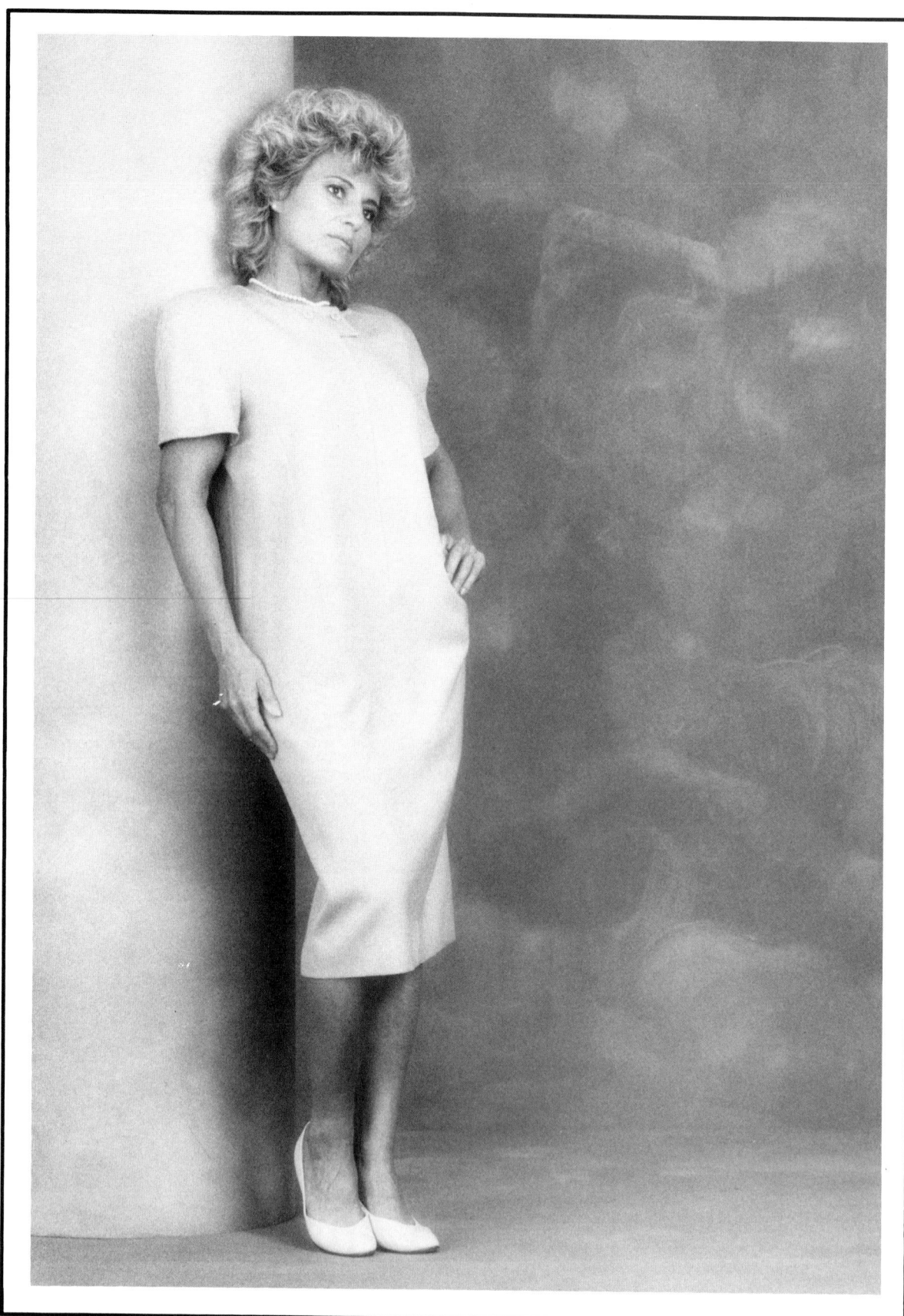

CHAPTER 1

THE TOTAL BODY LIFT

"I've tried everything. Nothing works. It's just another come-on. I guess I'll just have to accept the facts. When you get to a certain age..."

Wrong. You never have to accept a sagging body—drooping triceps (upper arms), falling, broadening buttocks, cellulite thighs, a protruding abdomen, and declining breasts. Not now. Not ever. And more important, you can begin today to reverse the gravitational pull on your body by developing muscles under now-sagging skin so that your body looks younger and tighter than it did ten years ago. In one year you can create a young, fit, firm body through the proven weight training program presented in this book, which takes only six hours a week. *Look at the "before" and "after" pictures in Chapter 11* to see the changes that are possible.

YOU CAN OFFSET THE AGING PROCESS

Everyone is subject to the gradual wear and tear on the body we call aging.[1] As we age, we slowly atrophy, or shrink. Each year after thirty we lose a small amount of muscle. We also lose a small amount of speed and strength. However, if we work to add on more muscle than we lose and if we practice to add speed, we can actually gain muscle and speed every year after thirty until way up in our sixties. It's true that athletes usually discontinue competition once they are in their thirties, because by then they have achieved peak condition and have no place to go but down. You, on the other hand, have not achieved peak condition or anything near it or you would not be reading this book. You have no place to go but up.

By building muscle, you can offset the aging process, firming up the muscles on your frame that time would otherwise wear down. Muscles serve as antigravity forces to keep your body from hunching over and looking withered. They also keep your skin from sagging, keeping it tight as a drum instead.

In the not too distant past, women were conditioned to believe that after thirty there was no place to go but "over the hill." Women such as Jane Fonda, Linda Evans, Cher, and Joan Collins have made this theory obsolete.

However, you are probably not able to spend the kind of time these women invest in their fitness programs. Fortunately that's not necessary. I have devised a no-nonsense body-shaping method based upon principles followed by champion bodybuilders that will deliver amazing results in three months. In less than a year you will have a perfectly symmetrical, hard, sensual body to rival that of any movie star.

The way I see it, the best years of life are the middle years. Youth is the time when one struggles with establishing her identity and goals and getting together all that is necessary to achieve the goals that are set. The middle years of life, from about age thirty to age fifty, are the years of flow, of peaceful movement toward goals. Having a beautiful body helps guarantee achievement. If you are burdened with a body that disgusts you, it is bound to set you back—in your career, your social life, even in your spiritual life. Much of your conscious and subconscious energy will be diverted by preoccupation with your dissatisfaction at how you look and feel. You will be sidetracked into worrying about minor issues when you should be free to deal with the major issue: *What can I do with the beautiful years I have left on this earth? What mark should I, could I make?*

HOW IT'S DONE

You might think achieving a vigorous, youthful-looking body in a short six hours a week is impossible. "How can I hope to develop a better body than movie stars who probably work out many hours a day and have private instructors—who knows, maybe even have regular cosmetic surgery?" you ask.

Simple. Through the carefully ordered use of weights, the only way such a body can be achieved. Aerobic programs help to condition the heart and lungs and help to burn excess fat. Some development of leg muscle is accomplished, but no overall reshaping is achieved. Tennis, racquetball, swimming, squash, volleyball—even calisthenics—cannot begin to reshape the body totally, replacing soft, sagging tissue with firm, shapely muscles. The only way to do that is to work out with weights. But working out with weights will not get the job done either if the weights are not used in the right manner and sequence.

Through years of interviewing champion bodybuilders, I have discovered workout secrets guaranteed to produce results. They have shared these secrets with me; I have used them myself to reshape my body totally and "lift" it into the shape you see now. The key is efficient use of the two principles of "pyramiding" and "split routines," which I'll explain in detail later (see pages 52–53).

As already mentioned, the only time investment is six hours a week, broken into four seventy-five-minute workout sessions and three twenty-minute aerobic sessions. You can fit these sessions into your busy schedule anytime day or night. That's the best part—you never become a slave to a set timetable for your workouts. You only have to be willing to invest six hours a week at your convenience to achieve a total body lift in one year. But you will see amazing results in just a few short months, and everyone you know will see those results, too.

Forget about Cosmetic Surgery

Yes, face lifts, "eye jobs," "tummy tucks," silicone implants, and the like do produce impressive results. Unfortunately, while such procedures do change one's physical appearance for the better, the results are not permanent; surgery must be repeated after a time. What is more, there is no way cosmetic surgery can implant muscle into every part of your body to give you the perfectly symmetrical and firm figure you long for.

But *you can* "implant" permanent muscle all over your body. By working intelligently with weights and feeding your muscles the correct foods (which are delicious), you can build a natural girdle around your abdominal area so that your stomach no longer protrudes. You can develop muscles all over your body to provide a frame that shapes your body and eliminates any sag in your skin. You will have tight buttocks, shapely thighs, firm breasts, attractive shoulders, and curvaceous arms. (Curves are really muscle lines, you know.) Your back will be that of an athletic woman. You'll soon look and feel better than ever before in your life—and better than many women years younger than you are.

Judy never worked out a day in her life until she was thirty-nine. At that point her body was one thin structure of cellulite. She looked beautiful in street clothing, but in a bathing suit she was an unsightly, spongy figure. Needless to say, Judy was rarely seen in a bathing suit. She was one of those women who believe in modesty at the beach, covering herself with a sundress every time she had to go to the refreshment stand. But after eight months of working out, her attitude had changed dramatically. "My body is completely transformed," she reports. "I try to show it off now whenever I can. It seems crazy that at my age I should be doing this, but I feel so sexy now. My teenage daughter is so impressed that she has begun working out with weights, too."

By working with gradually increasing weights you force your muscles to grow in size in order to meet the demands being made upon them. To give each muscle a chance to develop fully, you must force it to work in isolation. These are the two secrets of body shaping through muscle development: progressively pyramiding weights and muscle isolation.

How muscles grow to meet a demand is well illustrated by the example of Estelle, a school elevator operator. One day I asked her (knowing the answer in advance) why her right forearm and biceps were so much larger than those of her left arm. "You try and pull and push this heavy door all day long," she said in reply.

And none of us is surprised that construction workers have more muscle than the average office worker. Their job makes more demands on their bodies. But even construction workers often have misshapen bodies—beer bellies and skinny legs are common—because their physical labor does not require them to work all body parts equally.

So it becomes clear how muscles are "implanted"—by the demands of physical effort. Through following a careful, scientific workout program that involves all body parts, you can implant them all over your body naturally, without a bit of cosmetic surgery. You can do it inexpensively, and the results you get will be permanent.

Youthful Skin: A Workout Bonus

Women who have followed my program have not only achieved hard, tight bodies, they have developed vibrant, rejuvenated skin as well. Previously dry, limp facial skin has become moist and taut, giving the face a young, vivacious appearance. Barbara, one of the before and after examples in this book, is a classic example. Notice the difference in her face after just three months of working out.

It is because of the stimulation to the circulatory system that the skin is revitalized. In the course of a workout blood is pumped in greater volume to all parts of the body. Previously neglected, stagnant areas, including the face, experience renewal as a result of blood surging through them. (Another aid to youthful skin is drinking six glasses of water a day. We'll discuss this later.)

Why Working Out with Weights Often Fails

Five years ago I went into a high-priced, extensively advertised gym, and after a sales representative showed me around I joined. I was told to work out a certain way, using one machine for a quick exercise series and then advancing to another machine, or "station." This method, called "circuit training," was designed to improve lung and heart performance and give the body "tone." It does not provide the feeling of having worked hard on each body part.

I never thought to question why I was being asked to work on only one machine for my chest and then quickly advance to a shoulder machine and then a back machine and so on. I didn't know then that it is virtually impossible to reshape any body part unless you do *all* the exercises for that part in sequence. After working out as advised for almost two years, I finally became suspicious. No real change was taking place in the shape of my body. I did have a little more strength, and with a lot of flexing I could produce visible biceps. But that was not enough.

I wondered why I wasn't making the kind of progress I'd looked forward to. Not until I began writing for *Muscle and Fitness* magazine and became acquainted with world champion bodybuilders did I discover that what's crucial is not the time you put into weight training, but the order and sequence of the training. I discovered that body sculpting through weight training is an exact science. Once I began training according to the principles followed by the champions, it took only a year for my body to be reshaped into the perfectly symmetrical, dynamic figure I had always envisioned in my fantasies.

"Won't I Get Too Muscular?"

The most common fear expressed by women thinking of working out is that they'll wind up looking too much like a man.

Barbara had just gone to the gym for her first workout. She came home very excited, and then her husband said, "You'd better not get muscle-bound."

"How do I know I won't get too muscular?" Barbara asked me.

I reassured her that this would not happen to her. The workout program she would be following—the same workout program presented here—was designed to build shapely feminine muscles. There was no way it would turn her into a muscle-bound defeminized woman.

Perhaps you've seen pictures of gargantuan bodybuilders, both male and female, and worried that you could be transformed into their image. Stop worrying. In order to develop massive muscles like theirs, you would have to produce or ingest a hormone called testosterone in much greater quantity than your body is capable of producing it. Men naturally produce about ten times more testosterone than women. That is why men are more muscular than women (although exceptions do occur). In order for a woman to exceed her natural limits of muscle building, she has to take anabolic steroids—artificial testosterone formulations, which are usually injected. Steroids make women unnaturally muscular. Women who take such drugs (foolishly, I believe) develop unfortunate side effects—lowered voice, facial hair, genital malformations, and oversized muscles. They do begin to resemble men.

For a woman to become "overly muscular" without resorting to steroids, she would have to work out with extremely heavy weights twice daily, with a six-hour rest period between workouts. The women who do this are mostly professional bodybuilders seeking to become as muscular as possible in order to win bodybuilding titles. As you may have noticed, bodybuilders who compete in professional title competitions are becoming more and more muscular. To achieve that muscularity, they have to spend most of their time working out.

It is impossible for you to become "too muscular" as a result of following the routines prescribed in this book. You will certainly see muscle development, but it will be a natural development. That's what it's all about. Please welcome such development as you work with your body. Rejoice at the curves you are building into your figure. Enjoy your beautiful new sensual body to the fullest.

Two Fitness Fallacies Dispelled

If you want to take up the challenge of getting on with the real issues when it comes to total fitness, it's time to get your body under control. Don't settle for half measures. Scientific weight training is the only way to go.

Many women are sold on the idea that dieting will give them the body they want. It won't. Dieting alone cannot create muscles. Reducing your calorie intake can reduce body mass, but it cannot create muscle, nor can it firm or shape your body. That's why chronic dieters become so frustrated, even when they succeed in losing weight and move to a smaller dress size. They find they are still grossly out of shape. Dieting the wrong way can actually lead to muscle loss, and crash dieting with a binge aftereffect can result in a greater proportion of fat in body composition, even at a reduced weight. After a year of dieting, a dieter may find she is composed of little more than spongy fat despite being smaller in size.

Quit the group of lamenters who cluster around the cottage cheese and fruit salad, and join the adventurers who eat hearty meals of spaghetti, lean meats, all sorts of luscious fruits, and even "forbidden" foods occasionally. That diet you hope will turn you into a shapely, attractive woman by itself will only lead you to frustration.

Aerobics won't give you the figure you want either. The idea that they will is the second fallacy you need to clear from your mind.

Aerobics do have a positive effect. They condition the circulatory and respiratory system and somewhat tone and shape the legs and buttocks. But the upper body is not affected at all. Your chest, arms, shoulders, and back do not benefit. And your legs are not exercised in the correct fashion to form shapely muscle either. What muscle development does occur is "hit and miss." If you really look for complete body-shaping benefits, aerobics are not the exercises to concentrate on, although they do have their place. (I include aerobic exercises in my program. Their function will be discussed in Chapter 4.)

WHAT YOU CAN EXPECT FROM THIS BOOK

- A simple fitness program guaranteed to work if followed
- A completely new body in one year's time
- Self-confidence that carries over into career and personal areas
- The ability to use your mind to control your body
- Freedom forever from the fear of getting fat, soft, and flabby
- Release from the dread of looking and feeling old
- The physical strength to perform tasks you previously found impossible
- Freedom forever from torturous diets
- Freedom forever from the scale
- The ability and desire to help other women you know get into top shape, too

How This Weight Training Book Is Different

Most weight training books detail every possible exercise then propose complicated plans to follow using these exercises. Which exercises you do is left mainly to your own discretion.

In addition, most books require you to change your routine frequently, if not constantly. It is next to impossible ever to go on "automatic" so that you can stop thinking about what exactly it is you are doing and simply get on with it.

Finally, all other books put you on a time-wasting beginner's routine that will net you little or no visible results for months. I have worked with women for years, and I have found that they prefer to get right to the heart of the matter.

Forty-five-year-old Brenda told me, "The first day I worked out with your routine the gym owner asked me what I was doing. I told him I was following a routine given to me by my coach. He said, 'You can't do those exercises. They're too advanced for you. Let me give you a beginner's routine.' I refused, saying, 'I know what I'm doing.' I then did your routine, but only one set of each exercise, since it was my first week. When I walked out of that gym I felt terrific. The next day I was back. True, I was aching, but I loved it. I then proceeded to follow my Day Two workout for the other half of my body. The gym owner was amazed. Now [two weeks later] he's asking me questions, and he wants to know if I will train some of the other women who have been in his gym for months but shown very little progress."

In summary, we are not playing games here. I know that you have little time to waste. You didn't pick up this book because you are ecstatic about the condition of your body. You picked it up because you have considered or tried just about everything and you are at wits' end. Nothing has worked. You are clutching at your last straw. Well, I am going to make sure that it is the straw that saves your body, if not your life.

I will tell you exactly what exercises to do and in what order. I will tell you when to do them and how to do them. You never have to change your routine. You can work out this way forever and see continual improvement in your body. The only things you will ever change in your routine are the weights (when they become too easy to lift) and the repetitions (when you want to "bomb" certain body parts, say your buttocks and stomach), and these changes will be spelled out in simple language in the workout descriptions as necessary.

Because I want you to save your energy for the workout, I have done all the figuring for you. Your only job is to give it your best shot. A total body lift awaits you.

---

1. According to Dr. Gerald Feinberg, professor of physics at Columbia University, "Once an organism reaches the end of its growth, it remains on an apparent plateau for a long time, changing little in its overt functions. Yet even in this mature state, slow changes take place. There is gradual deterioration...this process is what we know as aging." (Gerald Feinberg, *Solid Clues*, New York: Simon and Schuster, 1985, pp. 124–125.)

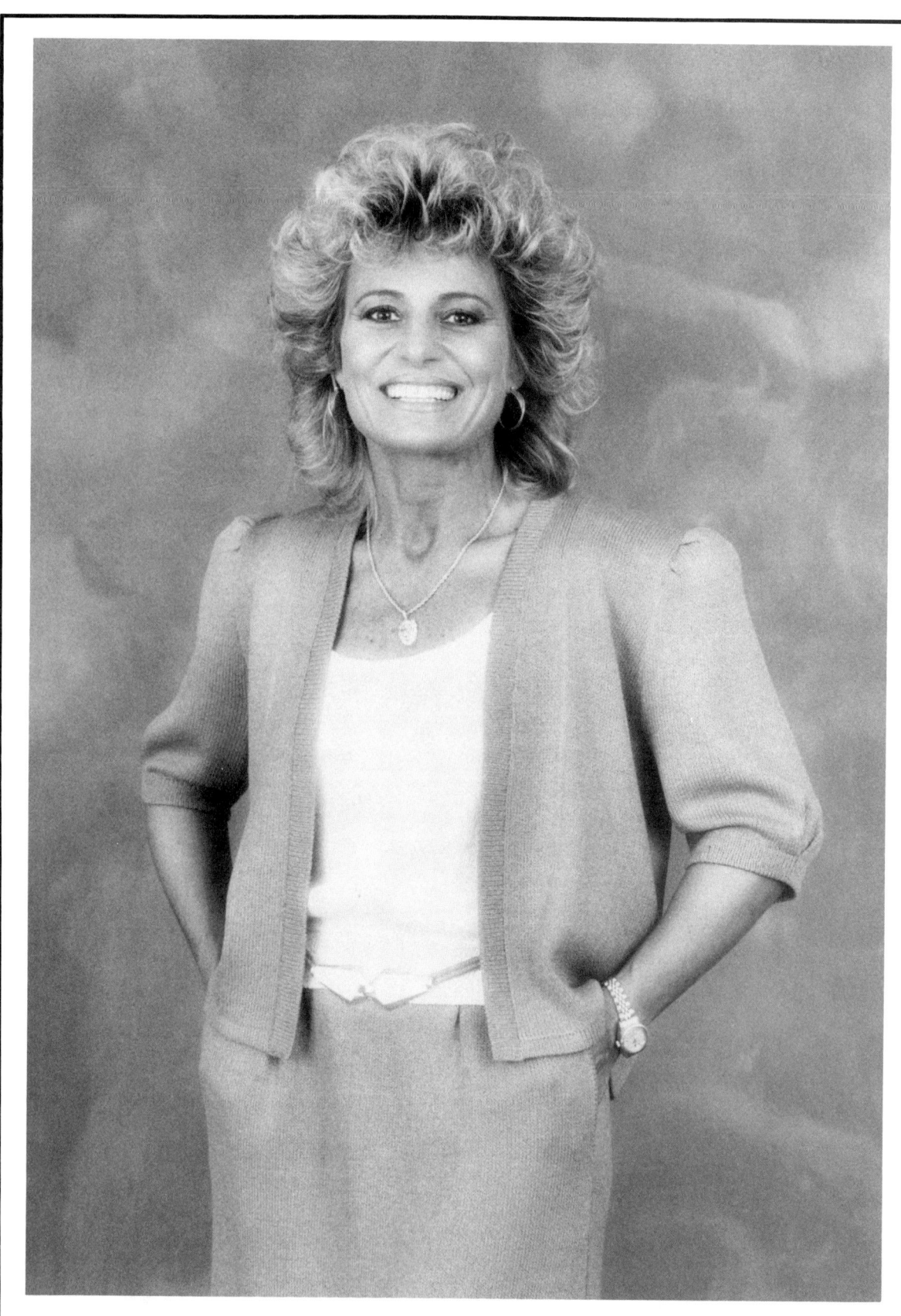

OUT OF SHAPE? LUCKY YOU!

CHAPTER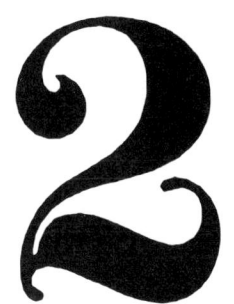

The way I see it, if you were already in perfect shape, you would be feeling a little depressed just about now. You would have no place to go but down. Top athletes face this problem and they are forced to retire from their careers. Their bodies have already achieved peak condition and every year (after about thirty) their bodies lose muscle and speed. You, on the other hand, are far from peaking. In fact, you have probably neglected your body, so have plenty of room for improvement. Even though you, too, are losing muscle and speed every year in small amounts, you will look and feel better and better as time goes on instead of worse and worse, because you are going to be putting on more than you are losing. So if you have a long way to go—if you are very, very out of shape—ironically, it is to your advantage. There's that much more room for improvement.

OUT OF SHAPE OR AGING?

Many people confuse aging with being out of shape. They assume that because a person has reached the age of thirty, forty, fifty, or older and is slowing down or looks as if he or she were beginning to "sag," that person is suffering from the inevitable signs of old age. In reality, even scientists cannot tell the difference between "old age" and "unused." "In the most carefully designed scientific tests it is virtually impossible to discriminate between the effects of aging and the effects of inactivity," says John Jerome in his book *Staying with It*.[1] "Much of what passes off as 'getting old' can be remedied by getting active."

You may have become victim to the idea that you are getting old, just because your life-style has forced you or at least lured you into an inactive life. Perhaps you have convinced yourself that what you look and feel like is the inevitable effect of getting older. You do not like this idea, but you accept it because you believe what you hear: "After a certain age..." "Stop trying to be a teenager." "Grow old gracefully."

Being Active Counteracts "Aging" Signs

When you become active, you pump blood through your circulatory system and stimulate your organs, bringing new life into them. Instead of atrophying and shrinking, your muscles keep working; they even grow. You "use them," so you do not "lose them."

One way to understand this simple principle is to observe the effect of wearing a cast on one's arm for six weeks. I recently had this experience. The cast covered my right arm from the elbow to my fingers—only the tips of my fingers were free of it. I continued to work out in the gym, "working around" the encased arm and doing whatever the cast would allow (and sometimes what the cast would not allow—I managed to wear away two casts by trying to bench press). When the big day came for the cast's removal I was horrified. My right wrist was diminished in size by about one-fourth, and my forearm was completely wasted. It looked like the withered arm of a ninety-year-old woman. I thought to myself, "I'll look like a freak from now on," but to my delight, it took less than five months for the arm to return to normal. In fact, it became stronger and bigger than the left arm. Evidently the neglected arm had a survival instinct that made it work twice as hard to get back to health, and it overworked. I actually had to force my left arm to work harder to keep up with the right arm after that.

There are two lessons to be learned here: What passes for or looks like the effect of old age may simply be the effect of lack of use, and a previously inactive body will respond quickly to stimulation, making gains in leaps and bounds.

WHAT ABOUT YOU?

Think of the muscles all over your body that you have never used or worked to any serious degree. No wonder you're now sagging and feeling withered and out of shape. Look at your triceps muscle (see the anatomy picture in Chapter 5 to pinpoint named muscles), the one located between elbow and armpit on your outer arm. Does that muscle wave back and forth when you move your arm? It's a favored evidence for people who like to show you how you're aging. The triceps is one of the muscles we neglect most because we don't use it much for daily chores. It remains tight naturally until about age twenty-seven and then begins to sag if one doesn't deliberately work it with weights.

Don't blame yourself if you have neglected this muscle—and most others as well. You didn't know better—until now. Be happy that you are finally learning a simple system you can use to transform your seemingly aging body into a young, attractive body. You will never again blame yourself for being out of shape once you use your energy to work those long-neglected muscles and watch them respond to the challenge.

I am delighted to say that it wasn't until I reached the age of thirty-eight that I touched a weight, and then I tried to use circuit training and didn't get very far. Not until the ripe young age of forty did I begin using the techniques described in this book, and by age forty-one I had a beautiful, shapely body. You can see the difference by looking at my pictures. I'm thirty-one in the "before" picture and forty-one in the "after" picture. I weigh the same (111 pounds) in each picture.

I had previously tried many physical activities, including the martial arts and excessive running, in vain attempts to get into shape. All these did for me was to develop hit and miss muscle. They did not get me a beautiful or young body. At the age of forty-two (my age in the cover shot and all other pictures taken expressly for this book), my body looks younger and more sensual as well as more symmetrical than it did even at twenty-five. And I was never really overweight.

Other women, like Roberta, have had to contend with a different problem. "Even at the young age of twenty-six I was a blimp, and I stayed that way until I finally started working out at forty-two. I feel ten years younger than I did when I was thirty-five, and as a matter of fact, people tell me I look younger." (Roberta is pictured on page 219.)

The Right Weight but Out of Shape

Perhaps like Judy, whom I introduced in Chapter 1, you look great in clothing but terrible in the nude. Your body is loaded with cellulite; you feel soft and spongy to the touch. You wear a size 10 dress and people compliment you on your figure, but you know you are out of shape even though you are not overweight.

Too Light in Weight and Out of Shape

You may even be what some people call skinny. Many women envy you because you can eat all you want and not get fat. You can wear almost anything, and with the right combinations of clothing you look elegant. Yet you look horrible in the nude—a combination of bone and loose skin and some fat. You are underweight *and* out of shape.

Too Heavy and Out of Shape

Or, maybe you are ten pounds heavier than you know you should be—maybe even twenty or thirty or more. You are fat. But if you think your only problem is losing weight, you are in for a surprise. Losing weight is only one of your problems. The other is getting into shape. You are overweight *and* out of shape.

Body Types

You may have heard of the traditional body types and wonder if you fit into one of those categories—endomorph, ectomorph, mesomorph. You do not. You fit one of the above descriptions. Body types are based upon the idea that people genetically fall into one of three categories—fat, skinny, or just right. Fancy names and descriptions are simply euphemisms that allow one to lean back and say "I'm a ___ type," and then have an excuse for not getting into perfect shape.

I discard the labels *ectomorphic* (lean and sinewy), *endomorphic* (bulky and tending to put on fat), and *mesomorphic* (muscular and nearly perfectly symmetrical). It is not because people do not *appear* to fit into these categories—they do. I discard the labels because by the time you finish working out with my program you will be "mesomorphic" anyway, and there goes the type. Furthermore, if you claim either of the negative labels (*ectomorphic* or *endomorphic*) as your type, you will be psychologically hindered from making progress. Subconsciously you will tell yourself that you are "fighting the tide." So forget about body types. Concentrate on developing yourself into the only body type that matters, your own ideal shape.

You and Your Scale— Muscle Weight or Fat Weight?

Another misunderstood element in fitness is weight. The scale is the instrument of deception here. It can only measure pounds; it cannot distinguish between muscle weight and fat weight. We've observed that an underweight woman can be out of shape. She may be light in weight but consist mainly of fat, which is comparatively light in weight. The ideal amount of fat on a woman is less than 20 percent. An underweight woman or one who is just the right weight may nevertheless have 35 percent fat. Since fat weighs less than muscle on a volume per volume basis, this woman may weigh less than a more muscular woman of the same height but look fatter. And her body will feel soft and unappealing.

Fat is made of a lightweight spongy material. It is airy and takes up lots of space for its weight. Muscle, on the other hand, is made of dense material. It is thick and takes up little space for its weight. Think of fat as a sponge and muscle as a piece of metal one-third the size of the sponge. The metal will *weigh* much more than the sponge, but it will take up less space. People who are muscular can weigh more than fat people and yet wear smaller sizes in clothing and look lean and in shape.

Pat, a forty-three-year-old travel agent, says, "I used to weigh myself every day. I would get so discouraged when the scale showed a gain that I'd go on an eating binge. Then the guilt would set in and I'd starve myself. Since I've been working out, I've learned to forget all about the scale. Now I only get alarmed when I see my body looking fat in the mirror. Then I watch my diet and work harder in the gym. In fact, I haven't weighed myself in who knows how long...I think four months."

"The only time I weigh myself," says Dolores, a thirty-six-year-old secretary, "is when I see in the mirror that I'm getting fat. But that's not a good idea because then if I do weigh myself and the scale happens to show a low

16 NOW OR NEVER

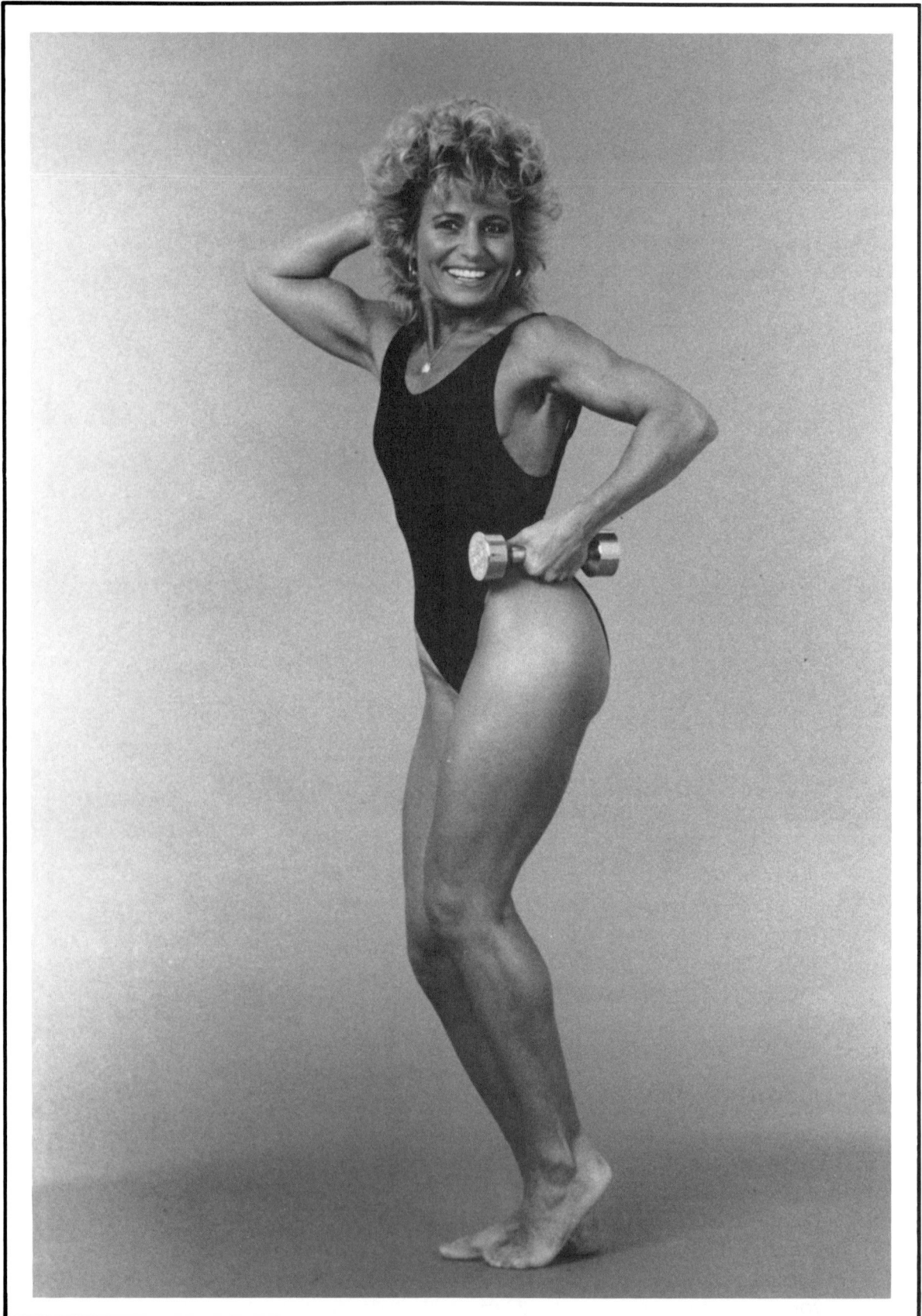

Photo by Bill Charles

weight, I tell myself I'm not fat and keep on eating. Then I get even fatter-looking, and eventually it shows up on the scale, too. Your best bet is to not use the scale at all."

If the scale tortures you, throw it out. In fact, throwing out the scale could symbolize your liberation from slavish diets and fruitless fitness programs that do not work. So, if it makes you happy, give it the old heave-ho. I dare you. You will not have to account for yourself by the scale. The program you are about to embark on frees you from that standard of measurement once and for all. You'll be using a new instrument of measurement.

Your Mirror as a Measuring Device

There is no question about it. What you see in the mirror is what you really are. I want you continually to look in the mirror and evaluate your progress. See if your stomach is too fat or just right. Let your eye determine whether your legs are too bulky and cellulite ridden or coming close to your idea of perfection. The mirror does not lie. Scales do. You can make the scale say you have lost weight. Most of us have done it—taken laxatives and water pills or not eaten for a day. The scale shows a loss, but in reality we look the same, or will the next day when the bulk and water return. We have used the scale to fool ourselves.

I am not forbidding you to weigh yourself. Just be sure to do so only as a curiosity—or because you are in the out-of-shape and overweight category (that is, you are more than ten pounds overweight).

WHAT IF YOU STOP WORKING OUT?

"I wouldn't want to be in your shoes ten years from now, when you can't work out anymore. All that muscle will turn to fat." Comments like this are typical of the misinformed, negative-thinking observer. Ignore them.

First of all, there's no limit on age when it comes to working out. And once you've watched this program produce results for you, you won't want to stop working out—not this year, not ten years from now. You will be addicted to the fitness habit.

Secondly, muscle does not turn to fat. It can't. Muscle merely shrinks back when you stop working out. Fat develops for other reasons. It accumulates on your body when you eat more calories than you burn through daily activity. When you stop working out, you lose the muscle and get smaller. Only if you take in more calories than you burn off will you get fat, and that doesn't have to happen even if you do decide to stop working out. I know. When I stop working out I get smaller and thinner, not fat. It's only the women who start working out at eating who get fat when they stop their exercise program.

Your Investment in Muscle

It may comfort you to know that every year you work out with weights is a year of muscle in the bank. It takes exactly as long as you took to put the muscle on to totally lose it. In other words, if you follow this program for two years and then totally stop, it would take two years to lose all the muscle you have gained from this program. If you worked out for five years, it would take five years to lose the muscle, and so on. But there is a bonus for you. It takes less than one-third as long to rebuild the lost muscle. For example, if you work out for two years then stop for two years and lose all the muscle, it will *not* take another two years to get it back again. It will take less than eight months to look the way you did after working out for two years the first time. You see, muscle tends to want to come back, and muscles seem to remember how to grow after having been taught the first time.

Kathy McBride, a thirty-two-year-old executive editor says, "I had stopped working out for two years because I had a baby. I returned to work but couldn't seem to find the time to return to the gym. I began to feel so out of shape that I couldn't stand it anymore. Finally I said, 'This is it. I have to make the time to do something for myself.' My baby had just turned one year old and I thought, 'If I don't do it *now* I'll *never* do it.' I went back to the gym and in one week I'm already feeling tighter and stronger. Even my walk is different—I have more bounce and people are commenting on it."

You can see then that working out is an investment for the future, no matter what happens.

Why You Won't Want to Stop Working Out

Working out becomes addictive. After three months you'll find you wouldn't give it up for love or money or even for your job. The only reason people stop working out after following this program for a while is injury or a life crisis. Those who are injured learn to "work around" the injury, doing whatever they can do, and those who experience a life crisis soon bounce back to working out because they realize that working out serves as therapy. "I come into the gym full of tension," says Maria, thirty-seven. "I leave feeling as if I had seen a therapist. All of a sudden I don't care about that problem. It isn't a problem anymore. Just a silly matter."

I asked some women what price I would have to pay them to stop working out. Andrea, thirty-five, says, "I have to be honest. I couldn't give it up. I don't think I could really stop even if you gave me a million dollars. I'd have no good feeling. What would I do?" "I would stop only if you would kill me unless I did—I'm not kidding," says Cheryl, forty-one. "Not for any money or anything in the world," says Marilyn, thirty-four. "How silly. There is no price on working out. It just can't be compared," says Dorothy, forty-three.

"Don't think about stopping. Think about starting. Begin the job and the work will be done."[2]

---

1. New York: Viking Press, 1984, p. 60.

2. Robert H. Schuller, *You Can Become the Person You Want to Be* (New York: Hawthorn Books, 1973), p. 92. Schuller is quoting Goethe.

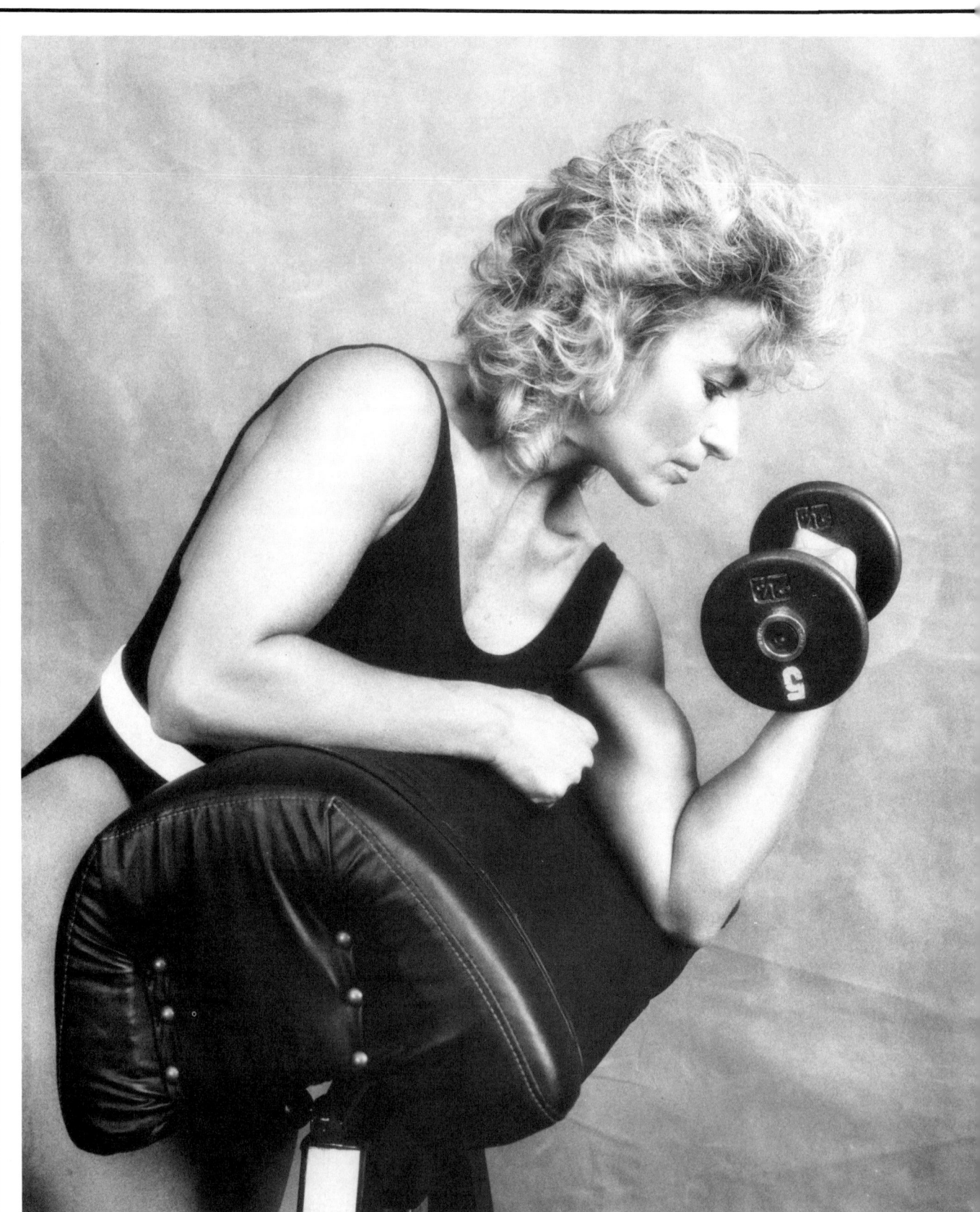

CHAPTER 3

WHO'S IN CONTROL—YOUR BODY OR YOUR MIND?

With maturity comes a calm. After a certain age, one tends not to see things as life-and-death issues or in terms of emergencies. Although those of us who have passed thirty-five do at times panic, deep down inside we realize that "this, too, shall pass," that if we maintain an inner balance, the answer to a problem will reveal itself.

This mentality is to your advantage as you begin the project of remaking your body. You realize that real progress cannot be obtained overnight, yet you know that results are achievable with constant intelligent effort. You have seen this principle at work in your career and in your personal life. You can call upon past successes in other areas of your life to help you. One step at a time and the goal is achieved.

At the age of thirty-five I climbed Mount Kenya in East Africa. The mountain is 17,500 feet high. I made the climb with a group of six people, and it took us three days. I recall looking up at the top of the mountain on the first day and wondering if I would really make it. But I did, and so did everyone else in the group—one step at a time. Then when I reached the top I looked down to the valley below and thought, "I don't remember climbing this great height."

You will look at your body a year from now and wonder how you were able to rebuild soft, flabby, "aging" tissue so totally into firm, shapely muscle. You will look at a picture of yourself "before," and wonder when the change actually took place.

THE MATURE MIND ACCEPTS GRADUAL CHANGE

Fad diets and quick shape-up programs are for the immature and the desperate. Such efforts, as you well know, end in failure and depression, with the addition of a subconscious confirmation that "nothing works." However, now that your own life experiences have shown you the reality of how change comes about, you have a distinct advantage over younger people who must still learn how change occurs. Those suffering from extreme youth must still pay the price of hard lessons learned from taking dead-end shortcuts. You have already learned those lessons. You are ready to use your mind to control your body and to help you to achieve the perfect figure you have probably fantasized about for years.

Now is the time. You have reached the most beautiful years of your life. The struggle of finding your career, establishing your identity, discovering your reason for living has already been waged. Now you can calmly devote your attention to perfecting your body.

YOUR PERSONALITY AND YOUR BODY

The body is the outer casing of the soul or the personality. When people first meet you, the first thing they see is your exterior, your body. If you are not happy with that body, you inevitably show it with an attitude of shame or apology. This cannot help but hinder your goals in dealing with people. You must once and for all get your body under control and out of your way. You must obtain for yourself a body that you are proud to present, a body that reflects your true personality.

Imagine yourself creating a body that would reflect your true inner being. What would it look like? Picture it in your mind. Look through magazines and find a picture of a woman whose body is similar to the one you feel would reflect your personality. This will be close, but your own body will be unique because no two people are the same.

I am a fun-loving, devilish person who is also very spiritual and sensitive. When I was thirty I had a body that did not reflect my personality. Now at forty-two my body says, "Athletic, strong, sensual, intense, exciting." I am now perfectly comfortable with my body. My body at thirty (ironically, when I was younger) said, "Lazy, discontented, bored, unhappy, disgusted, embarrassed, weak."

Find your true body-personality complement and resolve to transform your body into what you really are. Your mind will cooperate 100 percent because your mind, after all, is your personality.

YOUR BODY AND YOUR CAREER

If you allow your body to sag, become cellulite ridden, overly fat, stooped, or weak, you are sending out a false message about yourself to the world, and you will find yourself constantly trying to correct that false body message with verbal apologies. "I should go on a diet." "I've tried just about everything and I'm at the end of my rope." "Next week I start aerobics." "Oh, I can't eat lunch. I'm going to lose this weight if it kills me" (and it will). "I know I've gained weight since you saw me last. It was the holidays and then the..."

Many career opportunities can pass you by because you are forced to waste so much energy apologizing for your physical appearance. This continual apologizing detracts from your self-confidence, and you send out messages that you are not in control. People in power are often turned off to such a person. They believe that you are weak, because of the message coming through that you are not in control.

YOUR MIND CAN CONTROL YOUR BODY

In the past thirty years, psychologists have brought to light enough proof that the mind controls the body to make it clear that anyone who wishes to change his or her life is capable of doing so. There are cases on record of people able to accomplish feats way beyond their normal physical capabilities. A mother was able to lift a heavy truck off the back of her son, who was pinned under it, saving his life.[1] Her mind demanded that she do it. It was an emergency. Through the use of mind control, people can walk on hot coals without being burned. Others can accomplish amazing feats under the influence of hypnotism.[2]

What you believe about your capabilities directly affects what you accomplish. Vince Lombardi, former coach of the Green Bay Packers, says that winning is about 75 percent mental. "A man who starts believing he can win plays harder, stretches himself more, and helps those around him to do the same. He becomes more than he ever thought he was capable of becoming."[3]

You've got to start believing that you can in fact transform your body. Negative attitudes will not help you achieve your goal. As Nelson Boswell, a well-known positive thinker, once said, "Nothing can stop the man with the right mental attitude from achieving his goal; and nothing can help the man with the wrong mental attitude."[4]

Barbara Vale, Ellen Carter, Terry Perine, and Roberta Robinson had the wrong mental attitude. They believed that it was too late for them. But once they decided to believe, to say, "If others did it, why not me?" things began to change. You can see the results for yourself in Chapter 11. In this case a picture is indeed worth a thousand words.

I will show you how to use your mind to reshape your body. You will learn to control your eating habits as well as your workout techniques. You will learn how visualizing a perfectly symmetrical body leads to achieving that body.

Who's in Control— Your Body or Your Mind?

An "out-of-hand body," a body that has been allowed to run its own course, will take over your mind. It will cause you to feel lethargic and depressed. Perhaps you have been in the habit of listening to your body instead of your mind. Your body says, "Get up and get a few cookies and some milk from the refrigerator." Your mind says, "I really shouldn't." Your body then says, "Why not? You deserve it. You have nothing else in your life." So you listen to your body and you get the cookies...and then the cake...and then the ice cream and whatever else your body tells you it wants.

Now your body feels slightly nauseous and stuffed and extremely lazy. It tells you you can't get that job done tonight because you are really not up to it. Your body says, "Lie here and watch television awhile. You have a hard life. You deserve a rest." And your mind agrees, so that's what you do.

One example of the mind controlling the body is your reaction to an early morning ring of the alarm clock. Your body says, "Turn it off and go back to sleep." Your mind remembers a very crucial business meeting that morning, one that you have been anticipating eagerly. Your mind says, "No way. Get up immediately and prepare for that meeting. I want you to be sharp and on time." You get up and begin the day—end of conversation.

Why do you get up? Motivation. You had subconsciously prepared yourself to want to go to that meeting. Going to the meeting was important to you. You had already discussed that with yourself and decided to make sure you were there and at your best. Subconsciously you viewed the meeting as something that had to be done.

At other times you do not get up when the alarm clock rings. If you think about it, you prepared yourself subconsciously for that, too. You probably said to yourself the night before, "I hate to get up every day and go to work. I'm so tired of it. I deserve a day off once in a while." You may even have imagined yourself sleeping in without realizing that's what you had in mind. The quick mental picture of yourself not getting up with the clock probably passed through your mind in a flash. Then, sure enough, when the alarm rang in the morning you turned it off for another hour and called in late or sick when you finally did get out of bed.

YOUR TWO MINDS

Your mind is actually composed of two very distinct parts, your subconscious and your conscious minds. It takes both to ensure this program works for you. Harnessing the powers of your subconscious mind in support of your conscious resolve to change is the key to achieving your bodybuilding goals.

The first thing you must do is decide whether or not you love the idea of changing the body you now have into a dynamic, perfectly symmetrical, youthful body. You must make that decision before anything can happen. And then you must begin to believe that you really can make the change. After that your mind will cooperate every step of the way.

For years scientists and psychologists theorized that part of the brain specializes in imagery, creativity, and memory. They were convinced that one section of the brain recorded everything experienced by a human being, even as an infant in the cradle. However, it was a long time before they could prove this scientifically.

In the past twenty years, more has been learned about the human brain than in all of previous recorded history. We now know that the brain's two hemispheres, the right and the left, have specialized functions of their own. It is the left hemisphere that controls rational, conscious thought. It is the right hemisphere that contains what was previously spoken of only as the subconscious mind.

The Left Brain—Your Conscious Mind

The left hemisphere of the brain deals with logical sequences, numerical calculations, words and their meanings, and speech. It is the left brain, the conscious part of the mind, that plays the role of critic, commenting on everything you do. For example, when you are playing a game of tennis, it is the left brain that says, "You jerk! You missed the ball again. What's wrong with your timing?" The left brain makes no excuses. It sees only the details; it cannot see beyond the immediate facts. It knows only what is going on now, and it demands that things be in the proper order. It is scientific in approach.

The Right Brain—Your Subconscious

Your right brain, on the other hand, deals with whole pictures, images, faces in a crowd, putting puzzles together, creative thinking, intuition, and musical and artistic ability. Using the above example, it is your right brain that says, "So I missed the ball. I couldn't help it. I'm doing the best I can." The right brain thinks in terms of the whole picture rather than focusing on separate details. It "knows" things. It has what people call ESP. It is the right brain that processes information about an event or problem and comes up with "the answer," sometimes in the middle of the night, sometimes on a long walk, sometimes in the middle of an unrelated conversation. It works out the meaning or significance of details even though you may not consciously be dwelling on them.

USING YOUR LEFT-RIGHT BRAIN COMBINATION TO CHANGE YOUR BODY

You will find it easy to understand the complementary action of your right and left brains if you think in basic computer terms. Think of the left brain as providing the "input," or information that has to be processed in your mind. Think of the right brain as a natural creative computer designed to process that information in order to come up with solutions for specific situations or problems. Your left brain tells your right brain what the facts are and what the objective is. Your right brain examines the facts and works out the way to achieve the objective.

Reading this book is a left brain process. Through reading you accumulate the facts recorded here. Digesting the book and coming up with a personal application of this program to change your life through regular workouts is a right brain function.

As you read this book, tell yourself—your left brain "tells"; your right brain is "yourself"—to absorb the principles being presented. Tell yourself to believe that you can perform the simple mental and physical exercises presented here.

The input process starts even before you begin to work out. In order to reshape your body completely, you must identify your objective. Decide what you want to look like, and specify the changes to be made in your body. This is information your right brain must have in order to move you toward your goal. Once your right brain has this information input, it will act like a guided missile, zigzagging its way toward the goal you have set. (Maxwell Maltz and Dennis Waitley, among many others, provide countless examples of how this works.[5]) Once you set the program in motion by determining your goal, your right brain will automatically prompt you to make whatever corrections are necessary in your actions to reach that goal. You'll not only have made a conscious decision to change; you'll have harnessed the power of the world's most sophisticated computer—your subconscious human brain—to ensure that change comes about.

Visualization—the Input

Your first job is to get a mental picture of the body you wish to have. Stand in front of your mirror in the nude and look at the parts you want changed.

Picture your legs slimming down, shedding the cellulite and forming well-defined muscles. Picture your arms getting tight and shapely. See your shoulders taking form and your stomach flattening and becoming firm and defined. See your buttocks lifting and narrowing. Imagine your ideal body.

Stand in front of the mirror at least once a week and picture your body melting and re-forming into the perfect body. Tell your body (your left brain "tells") to get into that shape. Instruct your body to begin now to prepare for the program ahead. Notify it to be eager and happy to follow the workout and diet plan. Do this as mental preparation. Inform your body that in one year it will be perfect, that you will see gradual change every month. Be happy and rejoice in the fact that you have power to effect change. Do not let negative thoughts creep in. The negative thoughts come from the logical, critical left brain. Control your left brain input. Instruct your body to do as you say. It will. It must follow orders. It does not have a mind of its own.

USING YOUR MIND TO CHANGE YOUR DIET

In his book *Total Mind Power*, Dr. Donald Wilson comes up with a way to train yourself to hate foods that are bad for you and love foods that are good for you.[6] He suggests picturing a table filled with all the "forbidden foods," foods that tempt you but add unwanted fat to your body. Perhaps your list will include doughnuts, pastries, greasy chicken, sour cream, ice cream, french fries dripping with ketchup and loaded with salt, pork chops, etc. See yourself eating all of these foods until you are so stuffed you cannot walk away from the table. Imagine yourself feeling queasy and nauseous. Think of your stomach revolting against and your back aching from being so stuffed. Imagine your self-disgust, wishing you had never eaten these "poisonous" foods. Then change the picture. Visualize a table filled with nutritious, delicious foods—all sorts of colorful vegetables and fruits: carrots, peas, green beans, cauliflower, broccoli, peaches, pineapples, melons, and cherries. See lean meats: white-meat chicken and turkey, flounder, sole, and tuna seasoned to taste and smelling wonderful. See yourself selecting from this table the foods to satisfy your hunger and envision yourself getting up from the table with a shot of energy and a feeling of youthful vigor.

Spot Picturing

As often as possible, remind yourself that you do not like fried foods, red meats, sugars, and salt. Tell yourself (your left brain tells your right) these foods make you sick a few minutes after you eat them, that you really hate them. Tell yourself to be aware and alert, not to be tricked into putting them in your mouth before you know what you are doing. And tell yourself that what your body really loves and craves are the delicious, nutritious foods that contribute to its healthy growth (see the list in Chapter 9). Make this spot picturing a habit.

Laurie, a forty-year-old doctor, found herself drinking a bit too much. She had been working out with the program presented in this book for a year and a half and was in top shape, but she noticed that her drinking had advanced to five or six drinks on weekend nights, and at least a couple of drinks on other days during the week. Laurie tried this spot picturing technique, telling herself that when she drinks she gets headaches and that she realizes liquor in excess is poison. (Her original reason for trying to limit her drinking was that she felt herself "slowing down" physically. She was finding it hard to work out with the energy she used to have.) Sure enough, within a month after she began spot picturing, she had totally rejected liquor. Every time she tried to take a drink, something in her would repel it. She would not finish the drink. Without thinking about why, she would end up ordering a glass of club soda or diet soda. The drink would remain on the bar, and she would order another soda or two. Before long Laurie realized that she could no longer tolerate liquor. Now she finds herself able to drink once in a while, but only one or two drinks and those only on rare occasions.

Spot picturing works. It is a most powerful behavior modification method. Dr. Paul E. Wood, M.D., in his book *How to Get Yourself to Do What You Want to Do*, says, "As you practice and create in your mind the images of what you want to happen, the body gets the message to make the condition happen. Then the complex machinery of the biochemical and nervous system is set into motion and change begins to occur through natural physiologic process."[7]

In Laurie's case, her body actually began to develop an intolerance for alcohol, treating it like poison. A very real change took place.

Using Your Mind to Speed Up Your Metabolism

When you are overly fat, your metabolism slows down. Simply put, fat begets fat. The fatter you are, the less energy you burn, even while sleeping.[8] It has

30 NOW OR NEVER *Photo by Bill Reynolds*

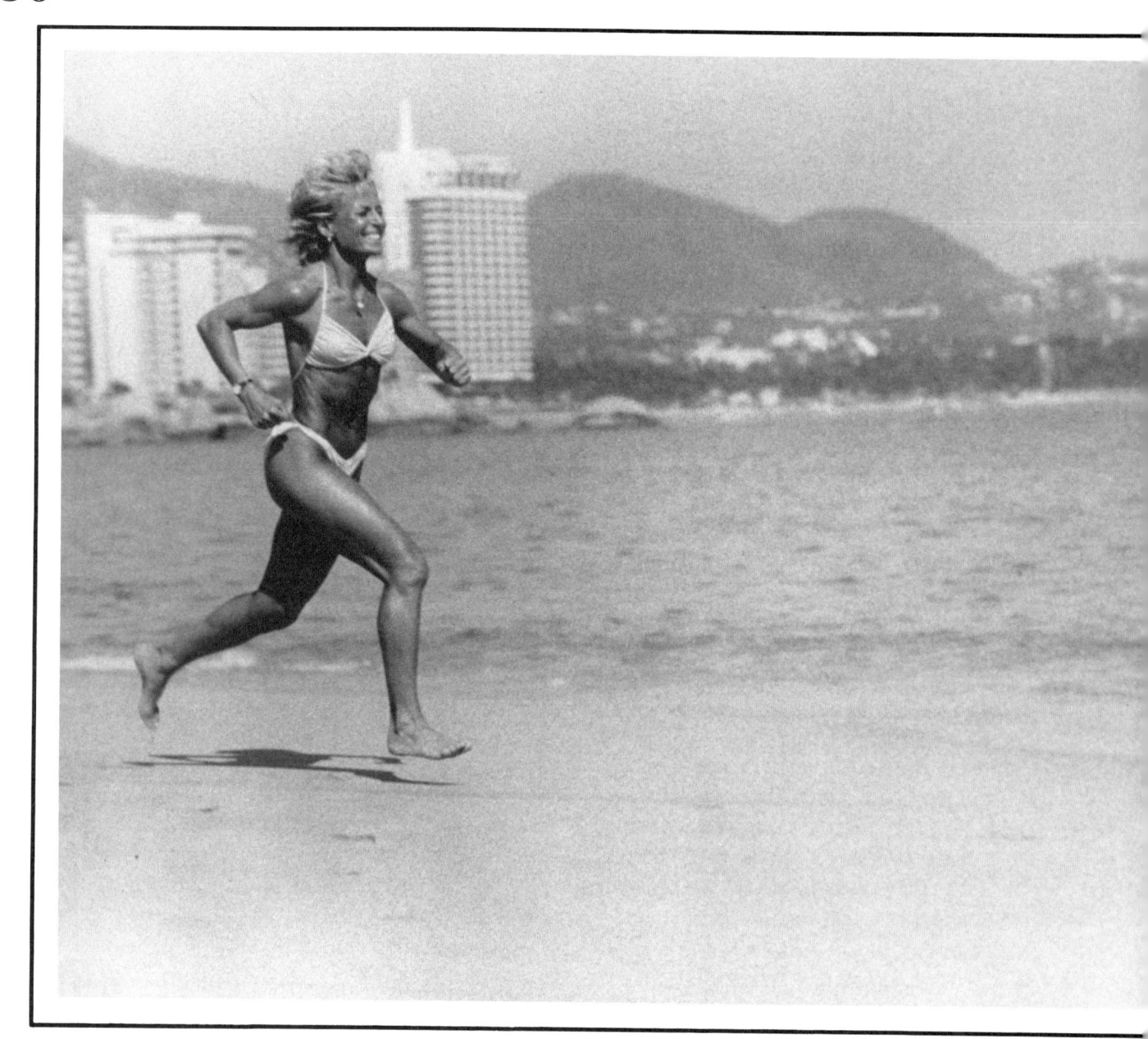

been proven that you can actually speed up a lethargic metabolism through mind control. You can make yourself burn about 20 additional calories an hour: Dr. Donald Wilson points out that there are specific areas in the brain which control the way food is metabolized. He tells his subjects to "turn on a switch" mentally, an "on" switch that steps up the metabolism. He tells them to do it every night before going to bed.[9]

I have tried this exercise and it works, not just at night but all day long. I find that it takes a few days before my body gets the message, but if I continually tell my metabolism to speed up, it does. I can literally feel myself tingling and burning energy just sitting in a chair. You should do this exercise if you feel lethargic and indolent. It really works.

Using Your Mind to Build Muscle

When you work out with weights, use your left brain to tell yourself (your right brain) to form the muscles into the shape you have pictured. As you work it, watch the muscle either directly or in the mirror. See it contract and expand; picture it filling with blood and growing as you work it. Tell your muscle to grow. Do each exercise in strict form. Picturing the muscle growing, telling it to grow, and doing the exercise in strict form are called "concentration."

A perfect time to spot picture is on the "flex" point of an exercise. For example, in the biceps curl, as you raise the weight to finish position, look at your bulging biceps and squeeze as tight as possible. This squeeze is called "flexing." As you flex, envision the muscle growing by a fraction and becoming more shapely and stronger. You will notice that we stress flexing, concentration, and visualization throughout this book. These three techniques can make you triple your progress. Remembering to concentrate, visualize, and flex will make all the difference in terms of speedy progress toward your body-reshaping goal.

Using Your Mind to Stay Young

Perhaps you have looked in the mirror and noticed another "line" or a gray hair and thought, "I'm going over the hill. It's only a matter of time before I'm old. And there isn't much I can do about it." Instead of accepting such thoughts and thus subconsciously allowing yourself to anticipate and welcome the signs of old age, resolve to detect such thoughts as soon as they begin to surface, and then repel them with immediate counterinstructions.

Cheryl, age thirty-six, used to think that she was hopelessly over the hill. Whenever she looked in the mirror at her shapeless, cellulite-ridden thighs, she told herself, "Oh well, you can't stay young forever. Leave the beauty contests to the younger generation." After learning about the left-right brain process she began to combat such thoughts with a positive counter-affirmation—"I can defeat this cellulite and reshape my legs. I still have lots of youth left. I'm not getting old until I'm eighty-five." She began to work harder and with more belief and now, a year later, she has no cellulite on her legs and people are taking her for twenty-six or twenty-seven. Looking back, she says, "I cannot understand why I was so willing to accept becoming an old bag way before my time. It was all in my mind. Why, I was actually welcoming old age."

When I see a wrinkle I don't like, or when I get a thought such as "You're beginning to sag," I immediately counter it with an input of energy. I tell my face to relax and rejuvenate. I tell my body to get tighter. I tell my subconscious mind my goal, and it achieves it for me. By accepting wrinkles and sagging I would be telling my subconscious to provide me a matronly carriage, a look I was rapidly getting at age thirty but which I have banished by right thinking and intelligent bodybuilding.

NEGATIVE THINKING VERSUS POSITIVE THINKING

Chances are some thoughts have been doing battle in your mind as you read this book. Perhaps you thought, "Interesting. Maybe I can actually do this." Then a contrary thought came in and said, "Who am I kidding? This is just another false lead. There must be a gimmick somewhere. What a fool I am to think I can do this." Then yet another thought comes: "Well, why not. It sounds logical. I like the way it's presented, so simply." Then a contrary thought again: "You can't do this. Think of all the other times you tried and failed. Don't make a fool of yourself by getting excited about another program. And by all means, don't tell anyone about it. They'll laugh at you and remind you of all the times you failed." Then another thought in answer to that: "So what if I failed lots of times. There's got to be an answer and maybe all the failures were leading to this—*the* answer." Your mind will go back and forth playing devil's advocate with you.

You are the only one who can determine which side is going to win the argument, the negative or the positive. Think of it this way: What have you really got to lose? If you try and fail again, you can still respect yourself for having had the courage to try, for not being a quitter. You can love yourself for your fighting spirit. You can congratulate yourself for being alive and in the ring till the last day of your life, never giving up.

And if you succeed (and you will), you will be preaching about the program to everyone you know, all the suffering beautiful women who are unwittingly slipping into premature old age because of wrong thinking and misguided fitness programs. Think of all the women you can help once you become a living example of what positive thought and action can achieve. You don't have to look or feel old at forty. (Even if you are not forty yet, you will be someday, and I don't want you to dread that day. You won't if you recognize your youthful potential and take steps to realize that now.)

Instead of worrying and thinking that you may not be able to do what is necessary to complete your goal of a totally new body, believe that you will achieve your goal. Wish it, pray it, believe it, run a movie of it in your mind. Do whatever you have to do. As Robert Schuller, the great religious thinker and philosopher, once said, "Prayer is worry turned inside out." Take your worry, your negative thought, and turn it into a positive belief, a prayer.

Never Verbalize a Negative Thought

Once you begin your workout, you may come upon an exercise that poses difficulty. You may catch yourself saying out loud to someone, "I'll never be able to do this."

Sandy, a forty-one-year-old bookstore owner, caught herself doing this. She was attempting a sit-up for the first workout day and could hardly get her body to rise more than a few inches from the ground. She said, "I'll never do this. Not in a million years." Then she remembered the detrimental effect that negative verbalization has, and she restated her point: "In a while I'll be doing this with no trouble." Immediately the expression on her face changed, and she did three full sit-ups.

The subconscious mind can't take a joke. Every time you make a statement, your subconscious mind registers it as fact. When you say out loud, "I can't," "I won't," "It's impossible," "I'm so clumsy," "I'm stupid," etc., your subconscious mind believes you and the task at hand becomes more difficult. You have created the additional obstacle of your unconscious to overcome. On the other hand, if you force yourself to restate your negative thoughts into positive ones, you will have added another helper to your inner support network. Now your unconscious will have on record as a fact that "in time I will be able to do this," and that silent affirmation will add momentum to your success in overcoming any difficulties at hand. So remember: *Catch yourself when you make a negative statement about yourself, and immediately change it into a positive statement.*

Younger Than Twenty

Women in their twenties and even younger are stricken with cellulite-coated bodies. Go to the nearest beach or pool and it won't be long before you see a young woman who has plenty of flab and a protruding abdominal area, and she may not even be overweight. Once you get used to seeing perfectly fit, hard bodies, you will begin to recognize out-of-shape bodies immediately. You'll find yourself thinking positively about yourself.

I wouldn't trade bodies with any person who does not use this program, not an eighteen-year-old, not a twenty-year-old, not anyone. My body is tighter, harder, more curvaceous than any young person who does not work out with weights. Your body can be the same and better.

A Year Is Not So Long

A year for a new body? But think of it. A year from now you'll still be here (God willing), and you'll either have the same unhappy body you have now, a worse body, or one that is perfect. Which is it going to be? Let's face it. The year will pass anyway. How will you feel then? Wouldn't you love to be able to look back a year from now, remember the horrible shape you *were* in, and congratulate yourself for the work you did to change your body? Wouldn't you like to have your body problem out of the way so that you can get on with your life? Wouldn't you like to spend your precious energy on things other than dieting and talking about being out of shape? And when you think of the changes you'll have made, a year isn't all that long a period of time, is it?

Go for It!

Emerson, the renowned philosopher, once said, "Do the thing and you will have the power." Take a chance. Try one more program. This one will work.

Go for it! Why not? After all, it's your life. You've got just so much left of it. Make the best of it. You deserve it, don't you?

1. Dr. Wayne Dyer, *Pulling Your Own Strings* (New York: Avon Books, 1977), p. 12.

2. Maxwell Maltz, M.D., F.I.C.S., *Psychocybernetics* (New York: Pocket Books, 1960), pp. 48–50. Dr. Maltz also discusses how self-hypnotism can affect a person's ability. He points out that we can either hypnotize ourselves to succeed or fail by continually telling ourselves that we can or cannot accomplish a given feat.

3. Nelson Boswell, *Successful Living Day by Day* (New York: Macmillan Publishing Company, 1972), p. 130.

4. *Ibid.*

5. Maxwell Maltz, M.D., F.I.C.S., *Psychocybernetics* (New York: Pocket Books, 1960), pp. 14–22; Irving Dardik, M.D., F.A.C.S., and Dennis Waitley, Ph.D., *Quantum Fitness* (New York: Simon and Schuster, 1984), pp. 25–26.

6. Donald Wilson, M.D., *Total Mind Power* (New York: Berkley Books, Inc., 1978), pp. 84–89.

7. Paul E. Wood, M.D., *How to Get Yourself to Do What You Want to Do* (New Jersey: Prentice-Hall, Inc., 1981), p. 90.

8. An average person burns around 60 calories an hour while sleeping.

9. Donald Wilson, M.D., *Total Mind Power* (New York: Berkley Books, Inc., 1978), pp. 82–83.

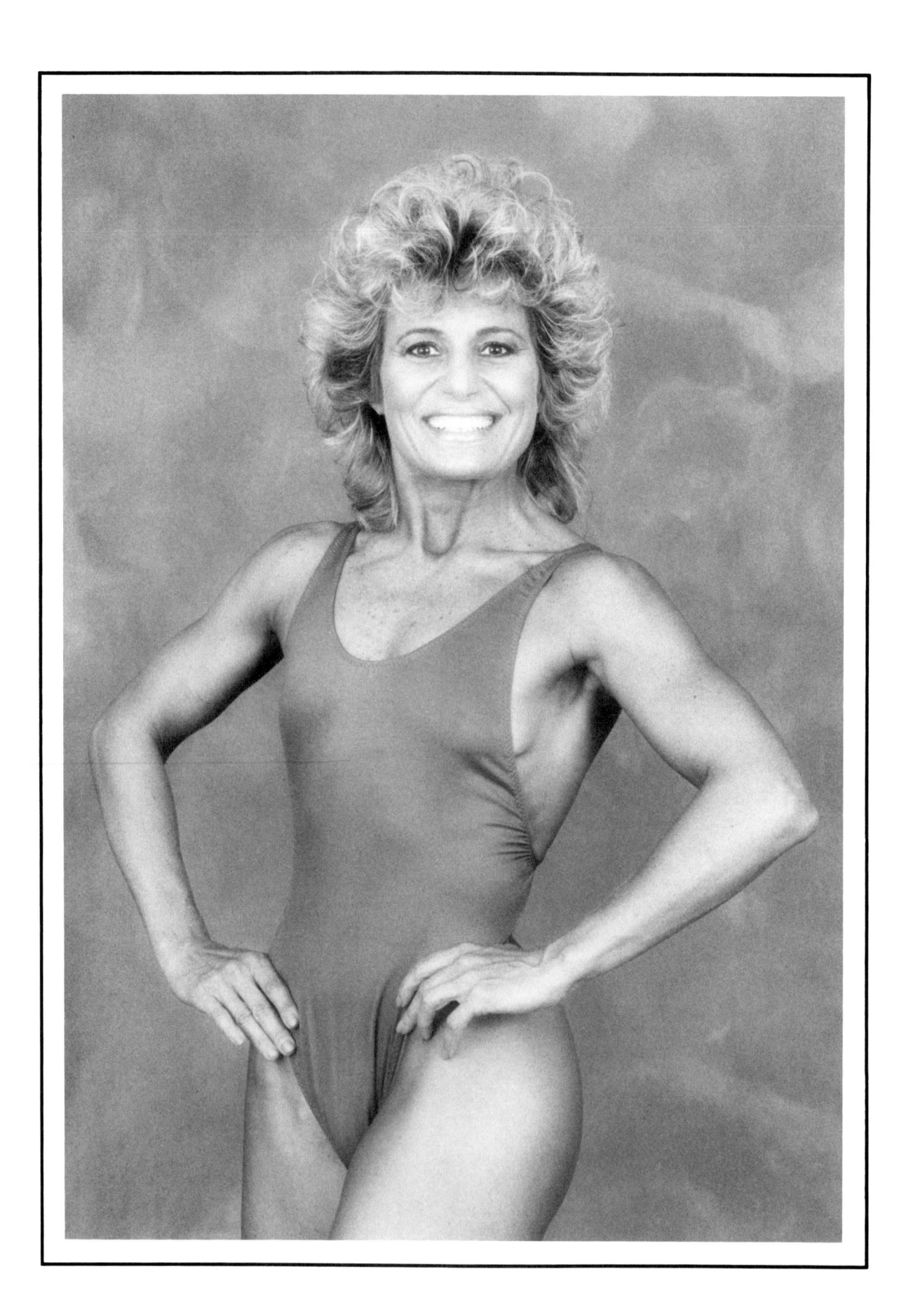

TIMING

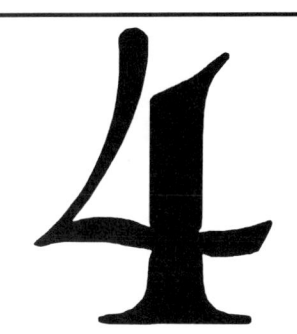

CHAPTER 4

This book is designed for women who have very little time to spare yet insist upon having an energetic and stunning body. It is designed for those who refuse to give anything up, for the women who want (and will have) it all.

Because of your very busy schedule, I have streamlined the program into six hours a week, broken up into four one-hour-and-fifteen-minute weight training sessions and three twenty-minute aerobic sessions. You will never be required to devote one minute more than that to obtain the perfect body, the "after" body.

FOUR WEIGHT TRAINING SESSIONS PER WEEK

It has been proven through experimentation that working a "split routine" four times a week gets the best results in the least amount of time for those who wish to obtain a perfectly symmetrical, hard, sensual body. Bodybuilding champions and their trainers have discovered and proven this, and I have successfully followed their training methods and taught them to other women.[1] The before and after pictures in this book show women who used the four-session split routine method.

Women who work out only one day a week find themselves in a state of continual soreness. When muscles that haven't been used for years are stimulated, they need regular exercise in order to break through the soreness barrier. Training only once a week does not provide enough stimulation to do that. As soon as the training day is over, the muscles lie dormant and return to their original state of weakness and lethargy. When after a week of rest the muscles experience new stimulation, there is new soreness. All that working out once a week does is serve to keep the body in a state of pain. It does not provide enough of a demand upon the muscles to cause any significant muscle growth.

With our program, working out twice a week stimulates all the muscles only once a week. This seeming contradiction is easily resolved when you realize that our "split routine" requires you to work only one-half of your body on alternate workout days. (This will be explained fully later.) Training twice a week while following a split routine will gain you continual muscle soreness for a reward of minuscule muscle development. The only real benefit of working out once or twice a week (if you don't mind the soreness) is the burning of some excess calories.

Bodybuilding three days a week would throw off our "split routine." The only way you could work out three days a week would be to work the entire body on each workout day, and experts such as Joe Weider, Arnold Schwarzenegger, Rachel McLish—in fact, every champion bodybuilder—will tell you that this is entirely too much work to do in one day. The inevitable consequence of this kind of overtraining is a poor workout and less than optimum results.

Women who do work out three days a week are probably utilizing circuit training, which is good for general toning and calorie burning but does little to reshape and create muscle.

Four days is the magic number. I train four days a week, and you see the results. At one point I tried training six days a week, reasoning, "If I can see such results with four days' training, I can look that much better training six days." It didn't work that way. I lost muscle size; I seemed to be working harder and getting less out of it. The most I can ever train is five days a week, and I do that only when I have the urge or I have put on some extra pounds and need the extra workout to burn calories. Working the muscles too much doesn't give them a chance to recuperate. They do not grow when they are overworked. Instead, they are worn down by the continual work and lack of rest.

If you follow my program and do the exercises in strict fashion, you will never have to work out more than four days a week.

Fitting the Four Sessions into Your Schedule

There are many possible game plans for getting the four one-hour-and-fifteen-minute sessions into your busy week. First choose the day that will begin your week. Sunday is a good choice since it is the first calendar day of the week. Choose any four days of the week from Sunday to Saturday as your workout days.

Since we are using a split routine, it will not really matter what four days you pick. You can pick Monday, Tuesday, Wednesday, and Thursday if you wish. It makes no difference. Most women tend to spread it out a little because they feel that it is less tedious to work out a day or two and then rest or do an aerobics session in between. This gives the body a chance to relax totally, and it prevents boredom.

I work out on Tuesdays, Thursdays, Saturdays, and Sundays. These days just happen to fit my schedule. I teach until 2:30 every weekday afternoon and work two nights a week until 9:30, so those times are out. I used to go to the gym in the late afternoon between my two jobs, but I found that I'd rather use that time to take care of other business on those days. Sometimes I am unable to work out on a Saturday because I have something to do with my teenage daughter, so I will get a workout in on Friday instead.

Your schedule is completely up to you. You may want to work out during your lunch hour—if you have enough time. Then again, you may want to go to the gym straight from work to avoid extra travel time and to sidestep the temptation to be lazy once you get home from work.

You may decide to work out before going to work. Many gyms are open early in the morning. If you are working out at home, there is no problem with this at all.

Some women like to go home from work and relax awhile, then get into gym clothes and work out, either in the gym or in their homes. Do whatever suits you.

Working out on the weekends is a matter of choice. Since I enjoy working out, I don't try to get it all over with during the week. I save some of my workout days for weekends, because I use that time to unwind.

The most important thing to do is establish a regular weekly routine and stick to it as much as possible. When something comes up, you have those three extra days to work with. Establishing a weekly routine helps you get the workout done. Deciding anew each week which days you are going to work out takes too much energy; it makes the workouts seem a burden. The idea is to fit them into your life in a natural, pleasant way, like taking a daily shower or a pleasant walk to the bus on a cool day. Before you know it, working out will become as natural to you as the simple daily routines you now follow, and as much a part of your life as they are.

Whether you are working out in a gym or at home doesn't matter. The important thing is to establish a routine. It is even more important to establish a regular workout routine if you work out at home rather than in the gym, because there are more distractions in the home.

AEROBIC SESSIONS

You must perform three twenty-minute aerobic sessions per week in order to condition your heart and lungs for your gym workouts and to burn excess body fat. Aerobics also give you an overall healthy skin tone.

Some women claim they can't do the aerobics exercises. They find aerobics too "boring." Barbara Vale (featured as a "before" and "after" in Chapter 11) was one of them. But after forcing herself to build up gradually from five to twenty minutes on the stationary bicycle she realized the benefit aerobics provided her. "You know, it's true," she recently admitted to me. "I find that I'm not as out of breath in the gym. I can go faster with my workout. There is definitely a carry-over. And when I started really doing the aerobics, I began losing weight more quickly."

Why Three Sessions of Twenty Minutes?

It takes a minimum of twenty minutes sustained aerobic exercise to achieve the optimum heart-lung stimulation required to maximize your body's responsiveness to weight training. You may increase the length of your aerobics sessions to thirty minutes and add one or two more sessions a week, but do this only if you want to burn off excess body fat. If you are too thin rather than too fat, do not do more than the required twenty minutes. I do extra aerobics only when I want to remove excess body fat.

Aerobic Choices

You may choose from a variety of aerobic activities. The favorites are: running, riding the stationary bicycle, jumping rope, swimming, and jumping on the trampoline. You may choose to walk instead, but if you do that you must double the time (that is, walk for forty minutes instead of twenty minutes), and you must walk unencumbered at a steady pace while swinging your arms. (Wear walking shoes or sneakers.)

I run or jump rope. The outdoors appeals to me, and I enjoy running even in the snow.

Other women prefer to ride the stationary bicycle. I notice that they are even able to read while doing so. Those who love the water enjoy a good swim for their aerobic session. I am a land person and would not venture into the water unless there were no other aerobic possibility. I once made temporary peace with the water when I sustained a torn cartilage from a judo injury, because I didn't want to interrupt my training. Nevertheless I returned to land as soon as the injury healed. (Swimming is the one activity allowed with almost any injury. For this reason it should be kept in mind no matter how much you dislike the water.)

Fitting in the Aerobic Sessions

I usually get the aerobic sessions over with in the morning. I find it a great way to start the day because, after a good run, I find that I have obtained a "natural high." I usually run Saturday and Sunday and two days during the week.

If I have had a late night and find it unwise to get up with only a few hours sleep, I will fit the aerobic session in later in the day. In this case I will probably jump rope in the evening while watching television or listening to a self-help tape.

Many women find that riding the stationary bicycle before a workout is both a natural warmup and a good way to get the aerobic session in. Others like to ride the bike after the workout because they want to save their main energy thrust for the weight training session and find it easy to ride the bicycle after the momentum of training has gotten them to full energy. I have run after a gym workout and found it exhilarating. When I run just before a workout I find it a little harder to pump the weights. To each her own.

It is wise to make a plan for the aerobic sessions just as you make a plan for the weight training sessions. You can alter your plan according to your needs, but a plan helps to ensure that you do accomplish the three twenty-minute sessions.

If you decide to do your aerobic sessions on your training days, you will have three days in the week to "do nothing." I don't think that is a good idea, because the body needs stimulation almost every day. It is better to leave only one day in the week to do nothing and to do at least two of the aerobic sessions on days when you are not weight training. Of course, I am speaking in terms of ideal situations. If your schedule calls for you to get the aerobic sessions in on your weight training days, no harm will be done. You simply may not feel as vibrant as you would have had you spaced them out more.

I have had to do all sorts of things to fit my workouts into my schedule, and I find that where there is a will there is a way. I find energy I never knew I had when my mind is set upon fulfilling my goal for the week, which includes working out, aerobics, teaching, business meetings, writing, socializing, family, etc.

SEEING RESULTS

You will feel results the first day you work out with the weights, but you will not see results for about three weeks.

The first week your muscles will be sore and "pumped." You will experience the soreness each day after training and the pump for an hour after training. The pump is a slight enlargement of the muscle caused by the increase of blood flowing through it as a result of the hard work being demanded of it. This pump lasts only an hour or so. The soreness lasts a few days. Of course, after a few weeks you will no longer feel sore.

The second week will be easier. You will start to get used to your routine. You will be doing almost a full routine and you will begin burning body fat. No visible muscle development will take place, but the changes are already beginning.

By week three you will be doing a full routine. You may see some slight definition beginning to show in your shoulder (deltoid) area. You may even see a slight rise in your biceps. Many women do not notice any increased development that soon, so do not despair if you see nothing. It is possible that you will, however, so don't think it is just your imagination if some change seems visible.

One Month

In a month you will begin to get used to your routine. There should be no real soreness, and you will feel an overall tightness in your body. Some body fat will have been burned, and you may see more development in your shoulder and biceps areas. Your abdominals may begin to tighten, and your legs will feel more muscular, but you may not see any noticeable improvement there yet.

Two Months

Everyone will see some body changes by now. Your biceps will show growth, a definite muscle development, even if slight. Your triceps will be tighter, and your shoulders will show definition. Some muscles will begin forming in your back, and you may see a line of definition in your thighs. In any case, they will feel tighter. Your chest will develop, too, a firm muscle beginning to form under your breasts.

Three Months

By now your buttocks will begin to lift. You will see they have narrowed, with well-rounded muscle forming under each part of your derriere. Cellulite will have decreased significantly. Your abdominal area will begin to form muscles, and depending upon how much fat you have covering that area, you will begin to see muscles forming and definition beginning to appear. Your breasts will continue to round out over the undergirding muscles, and you will notice that they stand out and are separated. This is caused by the developing pectoral muscles. Your shoulders will begin to have clear definition, and your triceps will show a tightening and also some definition. Other people will begin to notice that your body is changing.

Six Months

Your legs will show clear development. Your quadriceps or thigh muscles will form tight curves with pretty lines of definition. Your hips and buttocks will be shapely and tight. Your back will develop and your lattissimus dorsi, or "lats," will begin to take on the athletic V shape, giving your waist a smaller look. Your pectoral muscles will continue to develop, lifting and shaping your breasts further. Your triceps will no longer hang, and your biceps will be well formed. Your abdominal area will continue to tighten. Your overall body fat will have decreased; you will feel and appear tight and firm. People will begin remarking on the change in your body. Your clothing will fit differently. You will look for opportunities to show off your new body.

A Year

Now your entire body will have a new look. You'll stand straighter and look younger. Your walk will have a new bounce, and you'll have developed an athletic stride. Your chest will be firm and well-rounded, your breasts held higher by the pectoral muscles you have developed. Your shoulders will show front, side, and rear definition. Your trapezius muscles, which connect your neck to your shoulders, will stand out and give your neckline a flowing look. Your latissimus dorsi muscles will have created the V shape seen in swimmers' and gymnasts' backs, and your waist will appear smaller. You will have developed pretty muscles below your shoulder blades.

Your hips will be narrower, the excess fat gone, and your buttocks will be tight and well rounded because of the firm muscles you have placed there. Your front and back thighs will be completely free of cellulite, and they will have developed firm, well-defined quadriceps and biceps femoris (hamstring) muscles. Your calves will be well-formed, balancing out your thigh muscles. Your biceps will be well-rounded and very visible whenever you curl your arm or flex to show off your muscle. Your stomach will no longer hang out loosely, and there will be no fat to pinch. Instead you will have a line of definition going down the center of your body from your lower breast area to your navel. Your abdominal muscles will have developed, and you will see definition running from your lower abdominal area to your lower chest area. In short, you will have a hard, tight, appealing body that is close to perfectly symmetrical.

If You Are More Than Forty Pounds Overweight

If you are more than forty pounds overweight you may not see results in the time schedule described here. But don't despair. The muscles are being formed and are there, only they are hidden beneath the layers of excess fat. As soon as you drop below forty pounds overweight, you will begin to see the results as described. Remember: It doesn't matter whether you see the muscles or not. They are there. At least when the weight is gone, instead of having flabby, hanging flesh, you will already be in shape. The tight muscles will be there waiting for you.

Where Do You Go From Here?

Now all you will have to do is continue the program and perfect the stubborn body parts or those you wish to take a step further. ("Bombing" techniques for those who want to add finishing touches to their body are discussed in Chapter 10.)

---

1. Joe Weider, the founder of modern bodybuilding, originated the split routine as well as other bodybuilding techniques discussed in this book. He has been training champion bodybuilders, male and female, since 1945, applying scientific principles he first discovered. He is the owner and publisher of *Muscle and Fitness, Flex, Shape,* and *Sports Fitness* magazines and the sponsor of major bodybuilding contests. While you will not be working as hard as do the bodybuilding champions Joe Weider has inspired, you will be employing many of the same muscle development techniques.

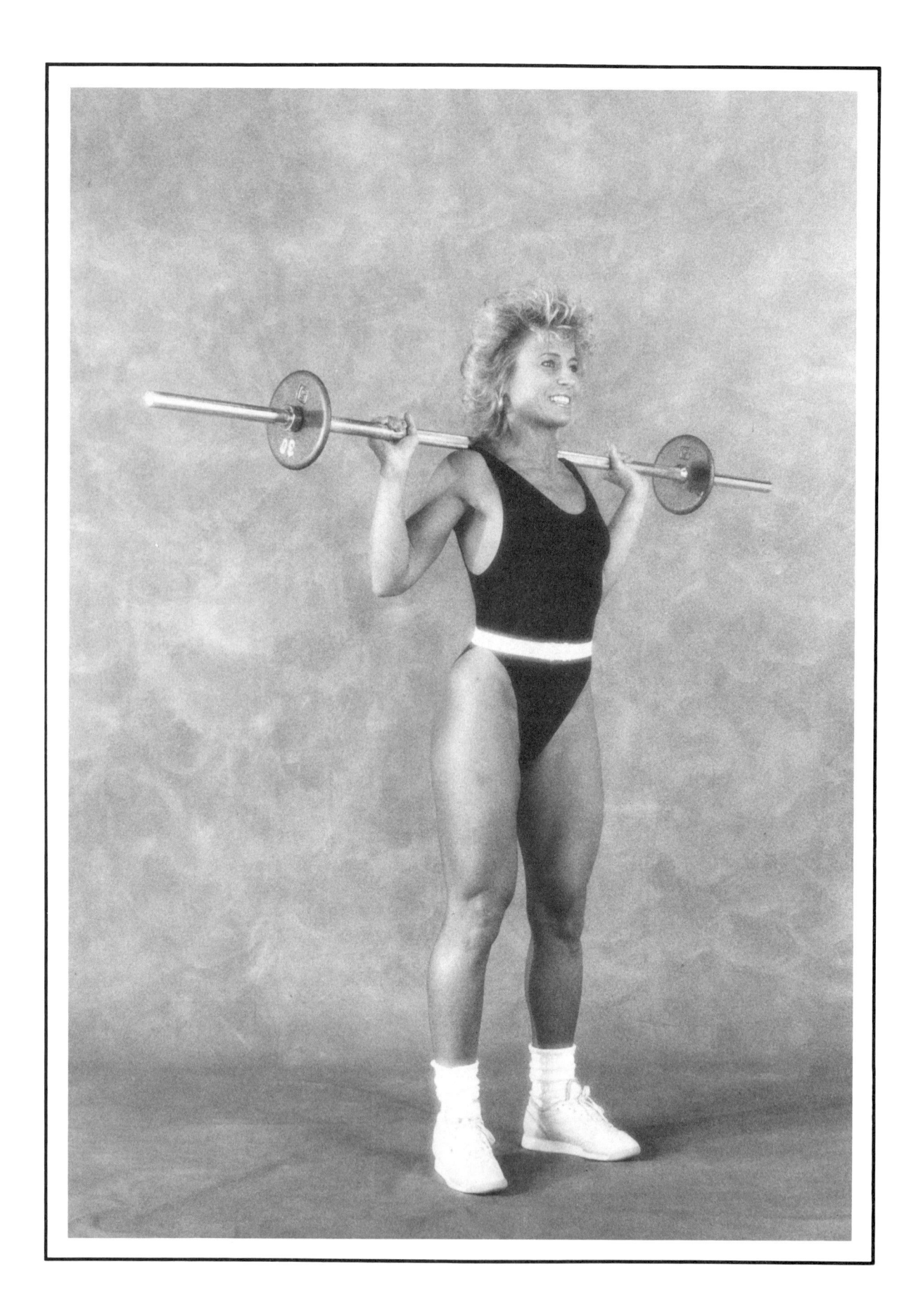

WORKOUT FUNDAMENTALS

CHAPTER 5

The workout program in this book is effective because you are required to isolate each body part and to work specifically on that area in exclusion of other areas. In order to understand what you are attempting to accomplish when you work a specific body part, it is necessary that you understand where it is located, what it is called both in common and "workout" terms, and what it does. Refer to the anatomy photographs so that you get a clear picture of each body part in your mind. Then stand in front of the mirror and locate each body part on your own body. Familiarize yourself with your own body so that when you are working out you can employ mental techniques to assist you. These techniques will be discussed later in this chapter.

48 NOW OR NEVER

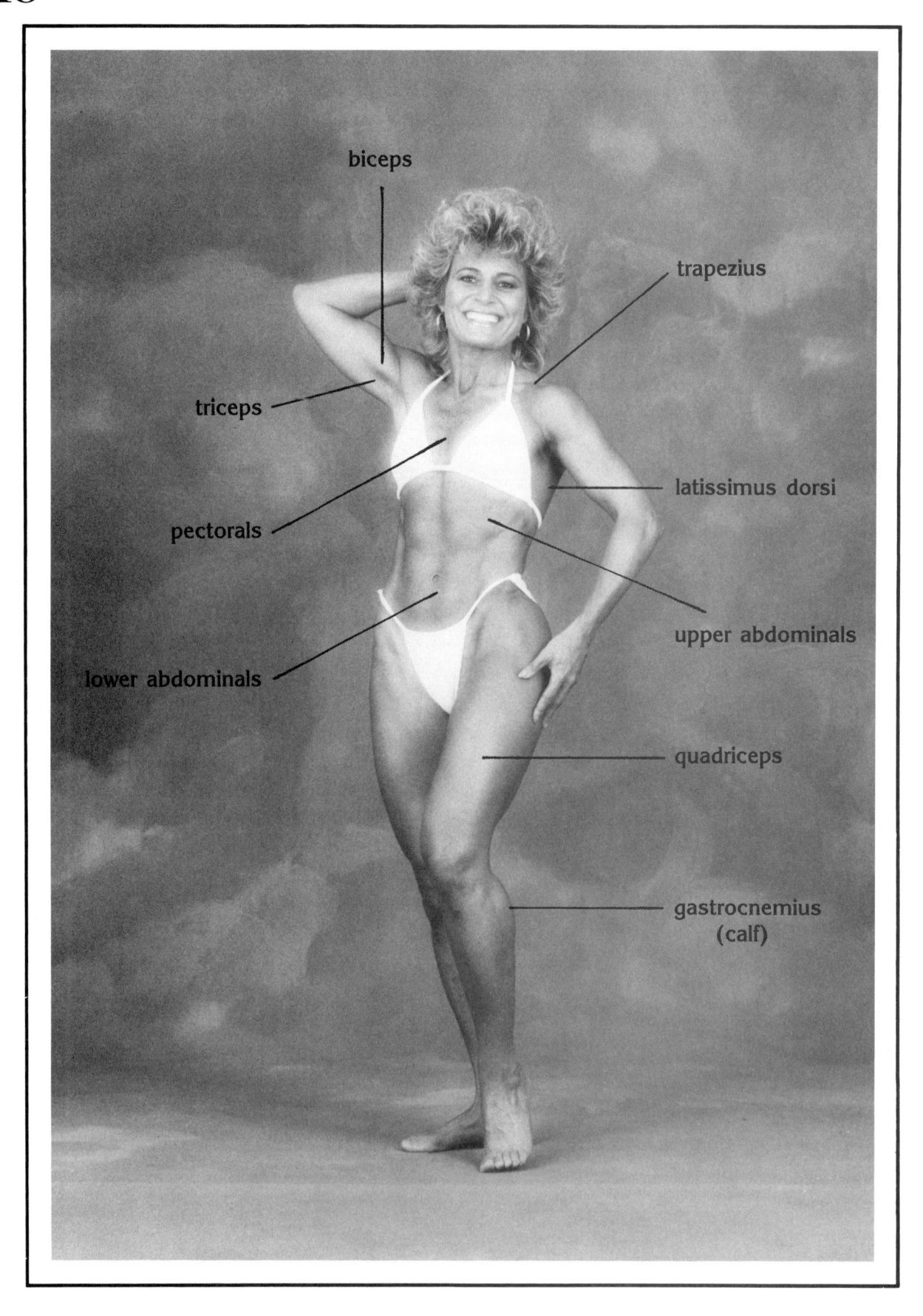

WORKOUT FUNDAMENTALS 49

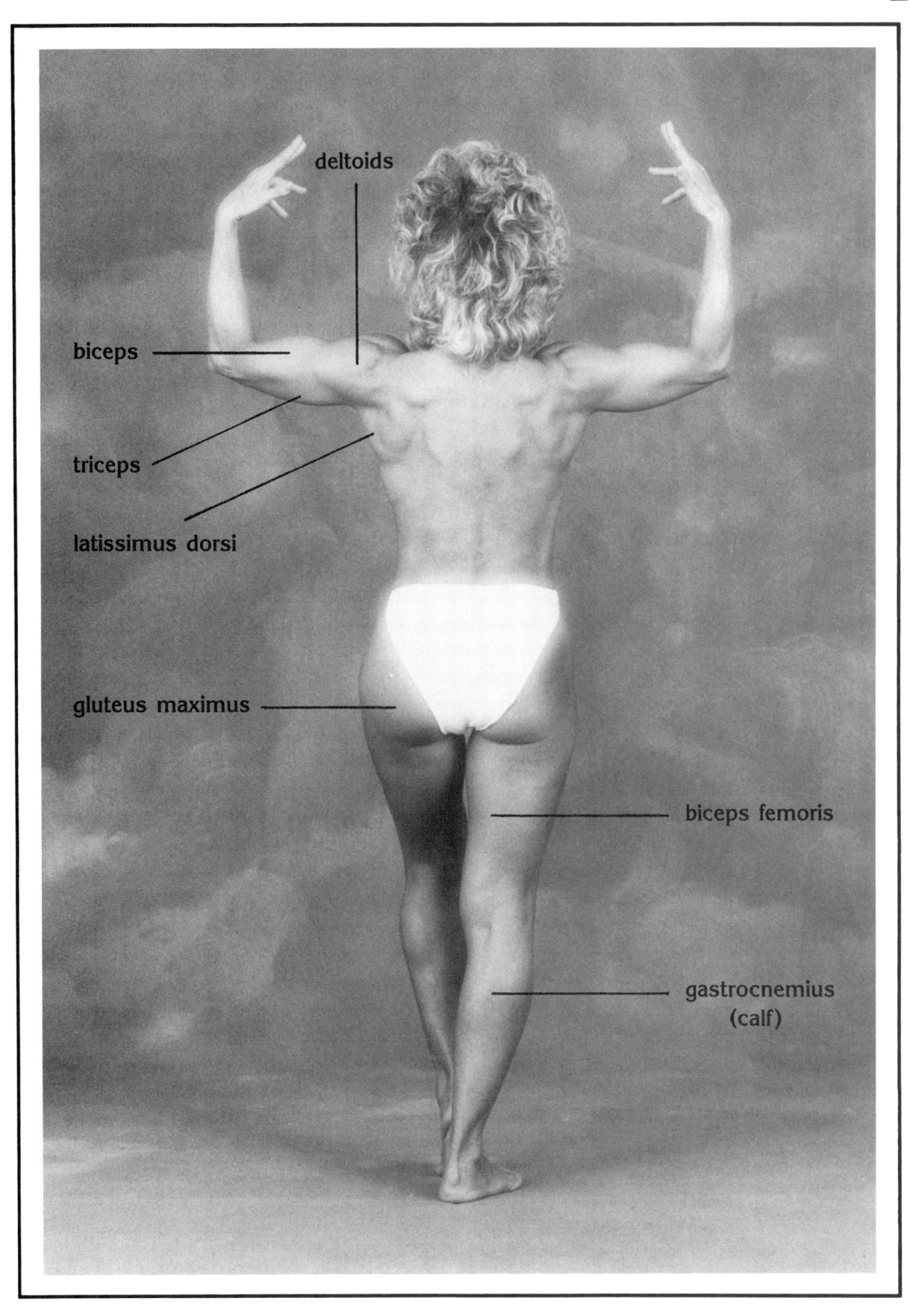

BODY PARTS

BICEPS. The large muscle in the front of the upper arm, located between the elbow and the shoulder joint, which flexes the elbow joint. This is the muscle used to show off when "making a muscle."

TRICEPS. The large, three-headed muscle (hence the term triceps) that runs along the back of the upper arm. It is used to extend the forearm. This is the muscle that sags if unused once a woman passes the age of thirty.

CHEST. The muscles located in the chest area are called *pectorals,* or "pecs." They are located in the upper anterior chest just under the breasts. When highly developed, they provide "cleavage." The pectorals are used in moving the upper arms.

SHOULDERS. The muscle that gives each shoulder its shape is the *deltoid.* This three-headed muscle helps to raise the arm. Although we speak of front, side, and rear deltoids, these are just different aspects of the same muscle.

BACK. There are two muscle groups in the back with which we are primarily concerned in this workout: the trapezius, or "traps," and the latissimus dorsi, or "lats." The *trapezius* muscles are the two large muscles running on either side of the spine from the back of the neck to the middle of the back. They are used to support the head and help to raise the head and shoulders and can be seen between the neck and shoulder area when developed. The *latissimus dorsi* rise along the spinal column from the middle of the back to the tailbone and give the back its greatest width. The *V* shape of an athlete's body is due to well-developed lats. These muscles are used to help pull the shoulder back and the arm toward the body.

ABDOMINALS. There are two abdominal areas that will concern us in this workout: the upper abdominals and lower abdominals. Both upper and lower "abs" are technically called the *rectus abdominus.* These muscles rise from the ribs near the breastbone. They help pull the torso toward the lower body and come into play in nearly every exercise. In Japanese and Chinese martial arts, the abdominal area is said to be the center of strength, the *Ki.* A strong abdominal area enables you to work harder at most other exercises. The "upper abs" are located from the waistline to the area just under your breasts, and the "lower abs" are located from the waistline to the upper thigh.

BUTTOCKS. The technical name for the buttock muscle is the *gluteus maximus.* This muscle is one of the largest in the body. It runs from the back hipbone to the tailbone and helps to extend and rotate the thigh.

LEGS. There are three areas of the leg, each dominated by a particular muscle: the front thigh (quadriceps), the back thigh (biceps femoris, or hamstrings), and the calf (gastrocnemius). The *quadriceps* is the large four-part extensor muscle at the front of the thigh. The *biceps femoris* ("hamstrings") is a two-headed muscle located toward the outer area of the back thigh. It flexes the knee, rotates the leg, and extends the hips. The *gastrocnemius* is the large, two-headed muscle in the calf of the leg and flexes the knee and foot downward.

UNDERSTANDING WORKOUT EXPRESSIONS

There is a certain "lingo" that exists in the bodybuilding world which one must understand in order to make workout life simple. This language consists of explanations of workout procedures, workout principles, and workout equipment.

Workout Procedures

EXERCISE. The actual bodybuilding movement being performed. For example, a barbell curl, used to work the biceps, is an exercise.

REPETITION OR "REP." One full movement of the exercise from start to midpoint and back to start again. For example, in the barbell curl, the raising of the weight from the start position of arms down to the midpoint position of arms up (curled) and back to the start position of arms down is one repetition, or "rep."

SET. A given number of repetitions. In this workout, your first set will consist of fifteen repetitions of the exercise. You will do three sets per exercise. Your second set will consist of ten repetitions at a higher weight, and your third and final set of the exercise will consist of six to eight repetitions at a still higher weight.

REST. The pause between sets (usually fifteen to forty-five seconds) that allows the muscle to regain enough strength to complete the next set efficiently. For example, in the biceps curl you would do a set of fifteen repetitions with a twenty-pound barbell and then rest for fifteen seconds. You would then do a set of ten repetitions with a thirty-pound barbell and rest fifteen seconds. Then you would do a set of eight repetitions at thirty-five pounds and again rest for fifteen seconds.

ROUTINE. The actual number of exercises performed by an individual for a given body part. For example, you will be performing four exercises for your chest. These four exercises constitute your "chest routine." In this workout, the four chest exercises are the bench press, the cross bench pullover, the cable crossover, and flyes.

WORKOUT. The entire bodybuilding session for a given day, made up of the total number of sets (including all body parts) performed. For example, on Day One, your workout will consist of routines for the chest, shoulders, back, abdominals, and buttocks. You will do twelve sets per body part, or sixty sets in all. (Don't worry. You will be breaking in slowly.)

Workout Principles

PROGRESSION. The gradual and continual addition of weight to the overall workout as the previous weights become too easy to lift, so that the muscles are continually forced to work harder and thus grow and make progress. For example, in the biceps curl you may begin by curling twenty pounds for your first set, thirty for your second set, and thirty-five for your final set. After two months you may find that you can curl the twenty pounds too easily, that you can do more than fifteen repetitions with no difficulty at all. You also find that, if you wanted to, you could do more than ten repetitions with the thirty-pound weight for your second set, and so on. The principle of progression demands that as soon as the weight you are using becomes of little challenge, you must raise it. You progressively increase your weight so that your muscle will increase in size, density, and strength.

PYRAMIDING. The adding of weight to each set of an exercise at the expense of a few repetitions. For example, in the barbell curl you may perform your first set with twenty pounds and do fifteen repetitions. Your next set will consist of a higher weight, say thirty pounds, but you will do only ten repetitions. Your third and final set will consist of a still higher weight, say thirty-five pounds, but you will do only six to eight repetitions. This is a modified system of pyramiding which has been proven to be the most effective way of developing maximum muscle size and strength in the minimum amount of time. A true pyramid would require you to perform two additional sets in reverse order, returning to your original weight—a set of reps at thirty pounds and another set at twenty to form a complete pyramid. Many champion bodybuilders recommend the modified pyramid for maximum results; most of them use this technique themselves. For the purposes of this workout, the term *pyramiding* will refer to the modified form.

SPLIT ROUTINE. The working of one-half of the body on one day and the other half of the body on the next workout day (except for the abdominals and buttocks, which are worked every day for special reasons to be explained later). Joe Weider discovered this principle in the early years of bodybuilding, and champion bodybuilders have been following it ever since. Spit routines allow the muscles time to recover and grow while resting, and they encourage the muscles to work up to capacity with strict performance during workout sets. In this program, your split routine will consist of the following:

Days One and Three
Chest, shoulders, back, abdominals, and buttocks

Days Two and Four
Biceps, triceps, legs, abdominals, and buttocks

You select the days, four out of any seven in the week.

Many women choose not to work out more than three days in a row even with the split routine, because they find their body rebels against a four-day-in-a-row workout. The most convenient way to break up your week, if your schedule allows it, is to work out two days, take a day off, and then work out another two days. It is important to note, however, that you will experience the same muscle development no matter what sequence of days you choose, because the split routine allows you to work out any day you wish.

Basic Equipment

FLAT EXERCISE BENCH. A standard-height bench that is long and narrow and padded, used to do exercises such as the bench press or the lying triceps extension.

INCLINE EXERCISE BENCH. A bench that can be raised to various degrees of incline (up to a 45° angle). It is required for exercises such as the incline flye or the lying incline dumbbell curl.

BARBELL. A bar upon which adjustable weights can be placed at each end. A barbell is held with both hands. Some barbells have permanently attached weights.

PLATES. Disc-shaped weights that can be added to either end of a barbell.

COLLAR. A holding device placed on either end of the barbell after a plate has been added so that the plate is kept in place.

DUMBBELL. A weight consisting of a short bar with a metal ball or disc at each end. Dumbbells can be held in each hand.

FREE WEIGHTS. Barbells and dumbbells. These are called "free weights," as opposed to "machines," because they can be carried freely about the gym, unlike machines, which are stationary. Many bodybuilders prefer free weights to machines because they allow complete control of the weight and force the individual to do all the work.

MACHINES. Nautilus, Universal Gym, Paragon, and a host of other machines specially devised for use in performing various exercises. Some machines operate on pulleys (e.g., Universal); others use cams (e.g., Nautilus). They provide variety for a workout. They also prevent injury, as they are able to "catch" the weight if you get tired and drop it while working out. For example, performing a bench press on the Universal Gym press would allow you to drop the weight, and it would automatically fall on the rack rather than on your chest. (However, there is little danger of free weights falling on you if you follow the simple procedures outlined in this book.)

I lean toward free weights but allow machines for variety.

Muscle Development

In addition to procedure, principles, and equipment, one must know something about the way muscle looks when it is beginning to develop. There are certain terms common in the bodybuilding world which describe the progress.

DEFINITION. When a muscle shows striations and sometimes a vein—when a minimum of body fat is present—the muscle is said to have definition. Another term for definition is *muscularity*. An example of definition can be seen in the washboard abdominal area of professional bodybuilders.

DENSITY. When a muscle is extremely hard it is considered to be "dense." Density implies a well-shaped muscle with total absence of body fat.

PUMP. Muscle expansion due to increased blood flow caused by the stimulation of repeated exercise sets. A pump can be seen in the biceps or chest for up to two hours after a workout before the muscle returns to its actual size.

MUSCLE SORENESS

Once you begin to work out, there will be a certain amount of normal muscle soreness. Ann, a forty-three-year-old mother of three, says, "I could hardly walk down the stairs. My legs felt like rubber. It was the strangest feeling. But I felt great. The ache reminded me that I was becoming strong. I loved it."

When you use muscles you have not used for a while or perhaps never used, it is normal to feel a dull ache of soreness. This pain is caused by microscopic tears in the fibers of the connective tissues in your body—ligaments, which connect bones to other bones, and tendons, which connect muscles to bones. When the slight tears occur, a swelling results because cellular wastes are produced. It is the swelling that causes the pain, but the swelling is too minute to be seen through the skin. When a real injury occurs (we'll discuss this later), the swelling is major and so is the pain. The swelling is quite apparent and must be treated with ice packs.

Ann's delight with her soreness is typical. There is a common workout "high" that comes with the awakening of muscles that have been lying dormant for years. The feeling is that of rebirth, and indeed it is a rebirth, in some cases a first birth of shapely muscles being implanted under sagging skin, muscles that will tighten the skin and cause the body to appear hard and shapely.

Many women ask whether or not they should stop working out until the soreness goes away. The answer is emphatically no. Continue to work through the slight discomfort, and in a few weeks you will wonder where the soreness went. It will happen so gradually that you will not remember exactly when it left. Maureen, a forty-one-year-old lawyer, reports, "The gym owner was surprised to see me back for the third straight day as he noticed me practically dragging myself up the stairs into the gym. He said, 'I thought you'd quit by now.' I thought to myself, It's a good thing I'm not relying on him for encouragement."

Maureen has the right idea. Self-determination is the key. Adopt the motto of triumphant bodybuilders: No pain, no gain. Remember, keep going. If you have a real injury, you will know it.

REAL INJURY

There is little chance of injury in the workout presented here. When working out with weights you maintain full control of the element you are handling: the weights. This is not the case in any other sport. Tennis players are at the mercy of where the ball leads them. They can easily twist an ankle. The same holds true for any ball sport. Those who participate in the martial arts are subject to their opponent's force. Only in bodybuilding can you totally control what is happening to your body.

Nevertheless, careless bodybuilding can result in injury. Not warming up at all, attempting to lift an extremely heavy weight for the first set, lurching with the weight or letting it drop, and ignoring correct form can result in injury.

This workout provides inbuilt insurance against every one of the above-mentioned dangers. A natural warmup is provided by the pyramid system, which requires that the first set be light enough to allow fifteen repetitions. There is a natural, gradual introduction to heavier weights with each subsequent set. Simple warmup exercises are also provided, and they only take five minutes so that women are not tempted to skip them altogether. The instructions repeatedly provide warnings about lurching, lunging, and dropping, so it is very unlikely that you will fall into sloppy techniques.

Types of Injuries

Certain injuries can occur, however, if one is extremely careless. A *fascia injury* can be incurred if one too suddenly jerks or pulls the weight. The fascia is the basic packaging tissue of muscles. When the fascia is torn, it becomes inflamed and the pain is severe. This injury must be treated with cold packs and wrapped in an Ace bandage.

Tendonitus, or inflammation of the tendon, can occur if you begin your first set with an extremely heavy weight and force yourself to lift or pull it even though that is almost impossible. This is a painful injury and must be treated by rest.

Ligament injuries can occur when an individual jerks or lunges too sharply. For example, if you jump into the lunge and land heavily on your knee, you may pull a ligament in your knee. This injury is treated with cold packs and a long rest.

Working around Injuries

It is never wise to stop working out completely when you sustain an injury. Continue to go to the gym and work whichever body part is not affected by the injured area. For example, a year ago I tore the tendon between my thumb and index finger and had to wear a cast from my elbow to my fingers. I managed to work every body part, including the biceps, which tie into that arm and hand. The only exercise I had real trouble with was the bench press, so I didn't do that one (after wearing away two casts). I increased the sets for my other chest exercises to compensate for not being able to do the bench press.

You may have an injury that causes you to stop working a body part completely. For example, if you sustain a ligament injury in the knee, you will not be able to work your legs at all. Simply work every other body part. A few years ago I tore knee cartilage. After a few months I was allowed to do therapeutic exercises for the knee. They turned out to be exactly my leg workout, except with light weights.

When you sustain an injury, that is a good time to "bomb" another troublesome body part. You can invest the time not being used on the injured part in a body part where you want to see faster progress. (See Chapter 10 for "bombing" techniques.)

Mental Control of Injury and Induced Healing

The mind plays a major role in the repair of injuries. Two people who are in comparable shape can sustain the same injury, and yet one's injury will heal quickly while the other's may linger, even worsen and eventually incapacitate that person. Why?

A host of psychological elements come into play when a person sustains an injury. Expectation of "the worst," a common reaction, certainly cannot help. It is natural to panic at first when you realize that, for example, you have torn the cartilage in your knee. Suddenly you are unable to walk normally, much less run, ride a bicycle, or work out in the gym. You may imagine never being able to return to full force again, thinking to yourself, "Once you pass a certain age, injuries don't really heal completely," or, "This is a sure sign that I am trying to fool myself into thinking I'm young again." However, when stopped dead with counterthoughts, that initial panic can do no damage.

The first thing to do when you sustain an injury is to accept it. It happened. Don't waste energy telling yourself, "I knew I shouldn't have gone to the gym today," or "This happened because I had an argument with my daughter." The thing to do now is make the best of the situation. In fact, make this seemingly negative event work in your favor.

After having accepted the reality of the injury, you must evaluate the seriousness of it. After getting a doctor's opinion, think in terms of working around the injury. Beware. Many doctors are overly cautious and will tell you to stop all exercise whatsoever. Another problem with doctors is that sometimes they will suggest that you have an operation for an injury that may well heal itself with time.

The important thing is your mental attitude. My philosophy is *Don't claim it.* For example, a few years ago I incurred an injury to my right knee. While standing around the gym where I was playing judo, a fellow judo player was catapulted onto my knee as he was thrown by his opponent. The pain was indescribable. The doctor immediately diagnosed it as irreparably torn cartilage. He even had the proof. He showed me an X ray of the knee and pointed out where the cartilage had been severed. He then fastidiously detailed to me how cartilage cannot heal and why it was necessary for me to have surgery. He reassured me that with the new method of orthoscopic probing I would not have to stay in the hospital very long. But then he said, "You will probably have to give up running for good." I will never forget what went through my mind at that moment. I mentally took all of his words, rolled them up into a ball, and threw them back at him. I said to myself, "I'm not claiming [accepting] this." I refused the surgery.

I then proceeded to limp about, first with an Ace bandage and crutches, later a cane, and finally with no aid, all the time touching my knee and telling it to heal. I pictured the torn cartilage and then pictured new cartilage growing. At night when the knee throbbed I touched it and massaged it, telling it to heal. I had faith. I believed my body had the power to heal itself.

The time arrived when I had to go back for a checkup. By now I was taking one-hour walks on the knee, and that week I had begun to run on it for twenty minutes. I'll never forget the doctor's amazement as he reexamined the knee. "What have you been doing?" he asked. I told him that I had been walking and running on it and going to the gym and working with the leg extension machine. He asked me how much I was running. "Three miles," I said, "but I'm working my way up to five." He put down his stethoscope, looked me straight in the eye, and said, "More power to you."

Don't claim it. Norman Cousins, renowned journalist and writer and author of the book *The Healing Heart*,[1] sustained a massive heart attack and was told that he would never function normally again. He was told that at age sixty-five his "myocardial infarction" (destruction of heart muscle) made this "fact." Not only did Mr. Cousins refuse to claim this so-called fact, he made a full recovery to function better than he had functioned before the heart attack.

Spurred by this experience, Mr. Cousins made it his business to discover the secret to healing itself. His studies show that the mind is 98 percent effective when it comes to recovering from an injury. He points out that the major reason patients do not recover in hospitals is their acceptance of the negative prognosis of the doctors. One of his simple experiments provides a graphic example of how the mind can affect the body:

> In the fall of 1982, I saw an ambulance in front of the clubhouse of one of the golf courses in West Los Angeles. I went over to the ambulance and saw a man on a stretcher alongside the vehicle. He had suffered a heart attack while playing golf. The paramedics, working systematically and methodically, were attending to their duties, connecting him to a portable cardiograph monitor, which they placed at the foot of the stretcher, hooking him up to an oxygen

> tank, inserting a plug in his arm to facilitate intravenous ministrations. No one was talking to the man. He was ashen and trembling. I looked at the cardiograph monitor. It revealed what is termed a tachycardia—a runaway heart rate. The intervals on the monitor were irregular. I also looked at the paramedics, who, true to their training, were efficiently attending the various emergency procedures. But no one was attending to the patient's panic, which was potentially lethal.
>
> I put my hand on his shoulder. "Sir," I said, "you've got a great heart."
>
> He opened his eyes and turned toward me. "Why do you say that?" he asked in a low voice.
>
> In Oliver Wendell Holmes's phrase, I "rounded the sharp corners of truth" with my reply.
>
> "Sir," I said, "I've been looking at your cardiograph and I can see that you're going to be all right. You're in very good hands. In a few minutes, you'll be in one of the world's best hospitals. You're going to be just fine."
>
> "Are you sure?" he asked.
>
> "Certainly. It's a very hot day and you are probably dehydrated. The electrical impulses to the heart can be disrupted when that happens. Don't worry. You'll be all right."
>
> In less than a minute, the cardiograph showed unmistakable evidence of slowing down of the heartbeat. The gaps between the tall lines began to widen; the rhythm began to be less irregular. I looked at the man's face; the color began to return. He propped up his head with his arms and looked around; he was taking an interest in what was happening.[2]

Norman Cousins has gone on to effect change in hospital treatment of heart patients because he has seen clear proof that how one thinks about an illness or injury makes all the difference.

In summary, you don't have to accept injury as permanent, nor do you have to "claim" the devastating effects so often predicted by well-meaning doctors. By a combination of mind and will you can be cured much more rapidly and with much less inconvenience than you could possibly imagine.

A final note on this topic seems apropos. I was telling people in the gym who sustain injuries to touch their injured areas and tell those areas to heal, reminding them to picture the injured body part mending itself. Around that time I received a book entitled *The Therapeutic Touch* in the mail from a book club, written by a nurse and Ph.D.[3] I read the book and, to my amazement, found there were a host of people who were one step ahead of what I thought was my own private healing discovery. As it turned out, Dolores Krieger had been teaching healing by touch and redistribution of body energy for a number of years, and she had gotten her program into major hospitals, where it has been proven to effect healing without medication, especially in babies. She now gives classes to doctors and nurses all over the United States who are employing the "therapeutic touch" or healing by the laying on of hands.

Thinking that Dr. Krieger's ideas might be rejected as unscientific, I continued to search for scientific proof that the body does indeed heal itself. I came across a new book, *The Body Electric,* by Dr. Robert O. Becker, an orthopedic surgeon, which describes experiments demonstrating that self-healing does take place.[4] Dr. Becker has proved, through years of laboratory experimentation, that injuries produce electrical currents stimulating the cells to produce new bone, muscle tissue, or whatever else is required to repair an injury. Now some doctors are using electrical stimulation to heal injuries.

I believe that we play a major role in assisting our bodies to heal and that we can touch the injury and stimulate the electrical current of healing by using the natural electrical current in the hand. It seems clear to me that we can assist our bodies to heal, and in time I believe the medical profession will demand more cooperation of patients in the use of their minds in lieu of reliance strictly upon "mechanical" treatments such as medication and operations for injury and illness. I believe, with Dr. Robert Ornstein, associate professor of medical psychology at Langley Porter Neuropsychotic Psychiatric Institute of the University of San Francisco, that our current knowledge of body energies may be compared to the knowledge of physics just before electricity was discovered, explained, and harnessed.[5]

THE IMPORTANCE OF CONCENTRATION

In order to get the best possible results from your workout, it is necessary to keep your mind on exactly what you are hoping to accomplish while working out. For example, if you are performing a lunge, rather than letting your mind wander into thoughts about what you are having for dinner that night, you must look in the mirror in front of you and watch your thigh muscle as it expands and contracts. You must mentally work along with the working muscle and tell it to exert itself and develop.

Concentration means "to bring to or direct toward a common center." In effect, you must direct your thoughts and energy to the common center of the muscle being worked. I have heard women say, "No one ever told me what this exercise is for. I didn't know the bench press was for your chest. I always thought it was for your arms." Such women are going through the motions and getting less than one-tenth the result out of the exercise compared to what they would get if they threw their mind and energy into the particular body part being worked. The woman in the above example, for instance, is probably thinking that she should do the work with her arms, so instead of stretching and squeezing (flexing) her chest as she performs the movement, she is pushing mainly with her arms. The end result is a poor workout of the chest and a haphazard stimulation of the arms.

Concentrate. I cannot stress this point enough. Continually think of the body part you are working, and direct all of your energy into that part. Always read the exercise instructions so you know what body part you are trying to develop. Keep your mind on that part. Pay special attention to the "Nevers."

They may at times seem repetitious, but they are very important. They will keep you alert to the natural temptation to cheat when your mind wanders from the strict form of the exercise.

It takes time to discipline yourself into concentrating fully. Don't be discouraged if you catch your mind wandering off to the business of the day. Simply forgive yourself for being human and bring your mind back to the exercise and the body part. In time you will find yourself going on fewer and fewer mental side excursions.

I must warn you of the most common way to lose concentration: talking to someone while you are working out. You will find that you must ignore everyone and simply give a friendly nod of recognition as you move through your workout. Most serious gym goers feel the same way (having learned through experience that talking can ruin a workout) and will understand that you are not being unfriendly. There is plenty of time for socializing after the workout.

Another way to break concentration is to waste time going for water or going to the ladies' room. Try to control yourself and wait as long as possible. Yes, it is true that water is good for the body, so I suggest you drink two or three glasses of water before your workout but then wait until you are finished and get another two or three glasses.

The final enemy of concentration is waiting. If you go to a gym machine or look for a dumbbell or barbell and find that piece of equipment is being used, move on. Go on to any other exercise in your routine for that body part. For example, your chest routine consists of the bench press, cross bench pullover, cable cross, and incline flyes. Suppose the bench press is occupied. Go to the dumbbells and get your first weight dumbbell for your cross bench pullovers. If that weight is being used, go on to the cable cross pulleys, and so on.

If you are on your last exercise, there is a gym courtesy others will usually extend you so that you don't have to wait: "working in." Virtually all bodybuilding gyms recognize and honor this point of workout etiquette. If an individual is using a machine, barbell, or set of dumbbells that you must use, too, simply ask if you can "work in." This means that when the other person finishes a set, you will immediately do your set, and when you finish yours, the other person will do his or her next set, and so on. No time is lost if you both quickly do your set the moment the other person is finished, because a set takes about thirty seconds and that is the normal resting time anyway. I don't like to work in because I normally take only about a fifteen-second rest between sets, and working in slows me down. Yet even I will work in when there is no other choice.

It's all part of gym survival. You are not working out because you have nothing better to do with your time. You are in the gym because you mean business. You have no time to waste on waiting around. Furthermore, too much waiting will negatively affect your workout. You have to keep moving in order to keep those muscles pumped and growing.

VISUALIZATION

As mentioned in Chapter 4, visualization involves mentally picturing what you want to happen. In a career situation, positive visualization might involve mentally picturing yourself responding spontaneously and intelligently at a job interview and landing the coveted position.

For workout purposes, visualization will involve you in two forms of mental picturing: body transformation in front of the mirror and muscle development in the gym.

Mirror Visualization

Stand in front of your mirror in a bikini bathing suit, in underwear, or in the nude. See your body as it now is. Now mentally resculpt your body into the perfect figure you have in mind.

Start with your top and work your way down. Look at your chest area. See your breasts being uplifted and becoming firm. See "cleavage" forming. See your arms becoming solid and your loose flesh tightening. See shapely muscles forming under your skin to form sensual curves.

Move on to your abdominal area. Picture the fat melting away and compact, tight muscles forming. See your stomach flat with delicate muscles forming a natural girdle. Picture the kind of stomach you've always dreamed about.

Move on to your hips. See the lumps melting away and visualize a narrow athletic-looking torso area.

See your back. Get a hand mirror and view your buttocks. See the excess fat and cellulite melting away. Imagine your buttocks being condensed, becoming rounded and tight. See the "wide load" look disappearing and the shapely, sensual backside of an athlete evolving.

Look at every part of your body and reshape it mentally. Tell your body to get into that ideal shape. Instruct it to do so within a year's time. Enjoy the thought that it *will* happen. When a negative thought assails you, wave it away. Simply see what you want to see.

If you have trouble visualizing your ideal body, look through fashion and exercise magazines and find a woman with a body something like the one you covet. You may look in *Shape* and *Muscle and Fitness* or other popular magazines until you find the body you have in mind. If necessary you can put together a body you want by combining the body parts of various women. Cut out the pictures and place them in a folder. Use them to help you in your mirror visualization.

Mirror-visualize at least once a week. Be sure to do it every time you happen to glance at your body when passing a mirror and a negative thought crosses your mind. Say you are passing the closet full-length mirror while wearing underwear. Perhaps the fleeting thought that goes through your mind as you catch a glimpse of your thighs is "Disgusting! Look at that cellulite." Immediately perform the mental exercise of imagining that cellulite melting away and the skin firming up. See a shapely muscle forming under the skin and fine definition coming into the thigh. Be happy at the thought of your progress. Then go on about your business.

Never allow your mind to dwell on negative images. Remember that it is your logical left brain "critic" who is pointing out the fault. Use your left brain instead to instruct your right brain to achieve the results you want. It is by mentally picturing the results you want that you give the right brain its instructions. As mentioned before, the right brain is a willing servant. You can put it on course like a guided missile to reach the designated goal. It has no choice once given direction. It is only a matter of time before you reach your goal—more time for some, less for others, but only a matter of time.

Visualization in the Gym

When you are doing a particular exercise, think about the body part you are attempting to develop and mentally picture that muscle growing and taking shape. For example, when you are performing the bench press, as you lower the barbell to your chest, visualize your chest expanding (you must do this mentally, because you cannot look at your chest, you must lie flat and look up). See the pectoral muscles fanning out and stretching. Imagine the blood flooding to the chest area. As you raise the barbell to starting position, see the pectoral muscles contracting, coming together, squeezing and pumping out the blood. Imagine your pectoral muscles beginning to get stronger, developing and forming into shapely mounds. You will find that as you visualize this way you will automatically stretch and flex your chest muscles as instructed in the exercise descriptions. The combination of visualization, concentration, and stretching and flexing speeds up your progress by 100 percent.

Naturally you will not be able to visualize every moment of your gym workout. However, even if you visualize one-half of the time, you will see amazing results in comparison to not visualizing at all. Learn to discipline your mind. In time visualization will become a habit.

TAKE A VACATION FROM LIFE

If you employ the methods of concentration and visualization, you will be forced to forget all of your troubles while you are working out. You will find that when you walk out of the gym, the issues that were on your mind before no longer seem as pressing. This is the therapeutic effect of working out. Many women claim that, for them, working out has taken the place of seeing a therapist. "I walk into the gym full of tension from my job," says Kathy, a senior editor of thirty-nine, "but by the time I walk out I am totally relaxed. Things that were irritating me no longer seem important. I think of simple ways to handle them, and I realize that I can work them out. Training really is a tension reliever."

The relief comes because you are unable to worry about problems while working out. This very short vacation from your problems serves as a "time away," and during that time your subconscious mind figures out simple ways of handling them.

TRAINING PARTNERS AND SPOTTERS

Whether you choose to work out in a public gym or a home gym, you will want to consider working out with a training partner. A partner need not slow you down if he or she moves quickly and does his or her set the moment you finish your set. A set usually takes no longer than thirty seconds, so if you instantly pick up the weight or get positioned on the machine and start your set you should waste no time. Since I work very quickly, a training partner invariably slows me down. I rest no more than an average of fifteen to twenty seconds per set. Most people take about thirty seconds to rest.

Aside from the possibility of slowing you down, a training partner can be a real asset. He or she can provide an incentive for you to push yourself when you are feeling weak or discouraged. In my gym I continually hear "That's it. You've got it. Two more reps," or "Tight legs. Go for it," or "Fight it. Don't give in." These are the voices of training partners spurring their comrades on.

Another advantage of a training partner becomes clear when you are trying to get in a last repetition but simply cannot find the strength to do it. At this point your training partner can give you just the slight assistance necessary to help you push your muscle a bit beyond what it would have done without the help. Without a training partner you would have to rely on whoever happened to be nearby, calling out, "Help me get this last rep." Chances are no one will be available.

A spotter can always be used in lieu of a training partner. Such a person can assist you to perform a difficult exercise by standing by and giving slight assistance. For example, when doing the military press, my last set requires me to press fifty-five pounds. Many times I have difficulty getting in the last two reps. When I ask someone to "spot" me (and I do this just before I lift the fifty-five-pound barbell onto my trapezius muscles in a ready position for the military press), I have no trouble getting in those last two reps. The spotter stands behind me ready to help me lift the bar. But not once have I actually had to use his assistance. For some strange reason, just knowing that he is there gives me that grain of extra confidence and energy to lift the weight for the last two reps.

Sometimes when the spotter does help, the help given is so minimal that the actual contribution is still almost purely psychological. Recently, a spotter helped me to lift the weights on my last, very heavy set of bench presses. When I finished I said, "You did most of the work." He replied that he had merely touched the weight. It was the thought that I had less weight to raise that made raising the weight suddenly manageable.

In summary, use a training partner if it suits your personality and needs. Use a spotter when you know you will have trouble getting in the last few reps of your last set.

---

1. Norman Cousins, *The Healing Heart* (New York: W.W. Norton & Company, Inc., 1983).

2. This selection is reprinted from "Antidotes to Panic and Helplessness" in *The Healing Heart* by Norman Cousins with the permission of W.W. Norton & Company, Inc. Copyright © 1983 by Norman Cousins. pp. 203–204.

3. Dolores Krieger, Ph.D., R.N., *The Therapeutic Touch* (New Jersey: Prentice-Hall, Inc., 1979).

4. Robert O. Becker, M.D., and Gary Seldon, *The Body Electric* (New York: William Morrow Company, 1985), pp. 146–147.

5. Robert E. Ornstein, Ph.D., *The Psychology of Consciousness* (New York: Harcourt Brace Jovanovich, 1977), pp. 132–133.

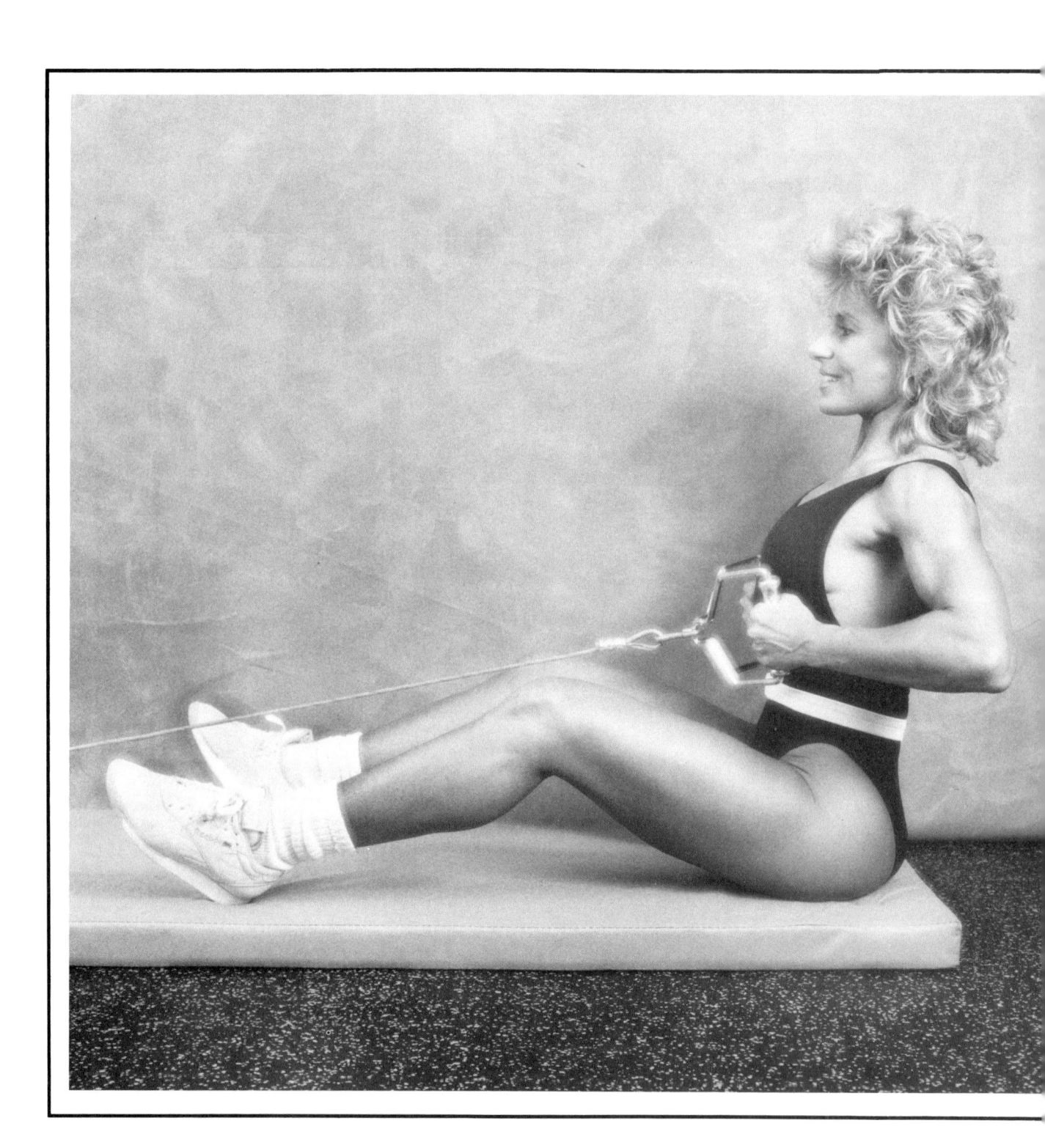

PREPARATION FOR BEGINNING

CHAPTER 6

In this chapter I will tell you exactly what you must do in order to get started on your routine successfully. I'll cover everything from warmup stretches to breaking into the workout slowly, then take you step by step through your first workouts.

WARMUP STRETCHING

Five minutes is all you need to invest in warming up. Begin by running in place for about thirty seconds. Next do ten jumping jacks. Then do five trunk rotations in each direction. Be sure to bend as far forward, to the side, back, and to the other side in your rotations as possible. Relax and flow with the stretch.

Next stand up and rotate your head, letting it fall first on your right shoulder, then your back, then your left shoulder, and then on your chest. Do three rotations in each direction.

Now, with your legs shoulder-width apart, touch your toes, using your right hand to touch your left toes and then your left hand to touch your right toes. Do three toe touches for each leg. Be sure to lock your knees for this stretch.

Lie on the floor and, with legs apart, sit up, lean over, and touch your head first to your right knee and then your left knee. Do this three times.

End your stretching routine by doing the bicycle for one minute. Lie on the floor and elevate your torso by placing your hands under your waist-to-buttocks area and move your legs in a circular motion as if you were riding a bicycle. Make the rotations as wide as possible.

That's it. Save the rest of your energy for the workout.[1]

BREAKING INTO THE WORKOUT—THE FIRST WEEK

Eventually you will be doing three sets of repetitions for each exercise, or sixty sets in all. If you were to try that on your first training day, you would be in so much pain that you might be tempted to quit. I'm giving you a way to start so that you will experience just the right amount of healthy soreness. The aches you will feel will inspire you instead of discourage you.

Training Day One

You will do only one set of each exercise. You will be working your chest, shoulders, back, abdominals, and buttocks on Day One. (Remember, we are on a split routine, working three body parts a day plus abdominals and buttocks, which are worked every day, for a grand total of five body parts every workout day.)

There are four exercises per body part. For the five body parts mentioned above, that makes a grand total of twenty sets (four times five equals twenty sets). Take my word for it, you can do that without danger of unbearable pain. Here is what you will be doing on Day One:

CHEST

Bench press—1 set
Incline flye—1 set
Cable crossover—1 set
Cross bench pullover—1 set

BACK

Lat pulldown to the back—1 set
Seated pulley row—1 set
Bent dumbbell row—1 set
Lat pulldown to the front—1 set

SHOULDERS

Side lateral raise—1 set
Front lateral raise—1 set
Military press—1 set
Upright row—1 set

ABDOMINALS

Straight board sit-up—1 set
Crunch—1 set
Bench leg raise—1 set
Leg-in—1 set

BUTTOCKS

Feather kick-up—1 set
Scissors—1 set
Back leg kick—1 set
Barbell tuck—1 set

You will do twelve to fifteen repetitions for each set. If you manage fifteen repetitions too easily, your weight is too light. Raise it (see page 75). Notice that when you count up all the sets they add up to twenty sets. By the third week you will be doing sixty sets in all, or three sets per exercise. However, don't think about that now. Take your time to break into the routine.

Training Day Two

Again, you will be doing only one set per exercise, but now you will be working the other half of the body plus the two parts you do every day (abdominals and buttocks). The body parts to be trained on Day Two are biceps, triceps, legs, abdominals, and buttocks.

There are four exercises per body part, except for legs, which require five, so on Day Two you will be doing twenty-one sets altogether. Eventually you will be doing sixty-three sets on Day Two, but that isn't until the third week, so relax. Here is what you will be doing on Training Day Two:

BICEPS

Standing barbell curl—1 set
One-arm preacher curl—1 set
Concentration curl—1 set
Incline dumbbell curl—1 set

TRICEPS

One-arm dumbbell triceps
    extension—1 set
Pulley pushdown—1 set
Dips between benches—1 set
Lying triceps extension—1 set

LEGS

Lunge—1 set
Squat—1 set
Leg extension—1 set
Leg curl—1 set
One-leg toe raise—1 set

ABDOMINALS

Straight board sit-up—1 set
Crunch—1 set
Bench leg raise—1 set
Leg-in—1 set

BUTTOCKS

Feather kick-up—1 set
Scissors—1 set
Back-leg kick—1 set
Barbell tuck—1 set

When you count up the sets they add up to twenty-one. You will do twelve to fifteen repetitions per set.

Training Days Three and Four

You will train with weights only four days a week. *On your third training* day you will *return to Training Day One and do exactly the same thing*. Do not increase your sets. Do only one set per exercise, or a grand total of twenty sets. *On Training Day Four,* the last training day in your first week, *do exactly what you did on Training Day Two*. Again, do not increase your sets. Do only one set per exercise, or twenty-one sets in all.

This completes your first week of training.

SECOND WEEK OF TRAINING

Now you are ready to do two sets per exercise. In other words you will be doing exactly what you did last week, only you will do two sets instead of one. This means that on Training Day One you will be doing forty sets in all instead of twenty sets, and on Training Day Two you will be doing forty-two sets in all instead of twenty-one.

Pyramiding Begins on Training Week Two

On Training Week Two you will begin to pyramid. You will do your first set as usual, with a weight that enables you to do twelve to fifteen reps. But for your second set, you will select a higher weight and do fewer repetitions—eight to ten. For example:

CHEST

Bench Press
Set 1.	30 pounds	12–15 reps
Set 2.	40 pounds	8–10 reps

Incline flye
Set 1.	8 pounds	12–15 reps
Set 2.	10 pounds	8–10 reps

Cable crossover
Set 1.	5 pounds	12–15 reps
Set 2.	7½ pounds	8–10 reps

Cross bench pullover
Set 1.	10 pounds	12–15 reps
Set 2.	15 pounds	8–10 reps

Because you are raising your weight, you must do fewer repetitions. Pyramiding causes the muscles to respond and grow, and it helps you maintain interest and feel challenged. In addition, the first set eventually serves as a warmup for the later, more challenging sets. Note: Under no circumstances are you to do more than ten reps for your second set. If you can do more than ten reps, your weight is too light. Increase it.

Do Not Pyramid Buttocks and Abdominals

The only two body parts that will never be pyramided are buttocks and abdominals. First of all, little or no weights are used when working those areas. Secondly, high repetitions are needed for all three sets when working those areas because of the nature of the muscles found in them. Your abdominal and buttocks areas are favorite places for the accumulation of fat. High repetitions with little or no weight are used to wear away the fat and stimulate muscle development in these areas. Do fifteen repetitions for each set. (You will eventually work up to twenty-five repetitions for all three sets—see pages 138–153.)

TRAINING WEEK THREE

This is the big week because it is the week during which you will do a full routine. Add one set to each exercise of your routine for a total of three sets per exercise. Now you will be doing a grand total of sixty sets on Training Days One and Three and sixty-three sets on Training Days Two and Four.

Full Pyramiding on Training Week Three

Now you are ready to do your complete workout and your full three-set pyramid per exercise. For example:

CHEST

Bench Press

Set 1.	30 pounds	12–15 reps
Set 2.	40 pounds	8–10 reps
Set 3.	50 pounds	6–8 reps

Incline flye

Set 1.	8 pounds	12–15 reps
Set 2.	10 pounds	8–10 reps
Set 3.	15 pounds	6–8 reps

Cable crossover

Set 1.	5 pounds	12–15 reps
Set 2.	7½ pounds	8–10 reps
Set 3.	10 pounds	6–8 reps

Cross bench pullover

Set 1.	10 pounds	12–15 reps
Set 2.	15 pounds	8–10 reps
Set 3.	20 pounds	6–8 reps

You may find that you simply cannot handle the next weight available in your gym in order to pyramid for your third set and that you must remain at the same weight for your third set. If that is the case, it's okay. No problem. Eventually, in about three weeks, you will get much stronger (I know it doesn't seem so now, but you will), and you will be able to handle the higher weight. That will be a landmark in your training. It will spur you on to work even harder. You'll feel really great about your progress.

For example, if you are doing the incline flye and your gym has only dumbbells that graduate from ten to fifteen to twenty pounds, etc., you may be able to get fifteen reps for your first set with the ten-pound dumbbells. For your second set, you may be able to get eight reps with the fifteen-pound dumbbells. But you may not be able to handle the twenty-pound dumbbells for your third set. Simply use the fifteen-pound dumbbells again and get six to eight reps for your third set.

You may have to struggle for the same eight reps now because your muscles will be taxed from the previous two sets, but push yourself. No pain, no gain. If you can't get the eight reps, six are okay because you're still within the allowance for your last set.

Your incline flyes may break down like this:

Set 1.	10 pounds	15 reps
Set 2.	15 pounds	8 reps
Set 3.	15 pounds	8 reps

HOW TO SELECT A BEGINNING WEIGHT

When you enter the gym with this book in hand and approach the first exercise, you may be wondering how to determine which weight to begin with. Simply select a very light weight and test it out. For example, your first exercise is the bench press. You should try to press as light as twenty pounds. If you get fifteen repetitions easily with the twenty-pound weight, that is fine for starters because you are breaking into the exercise. However, if it is so ridiculously easy that you feel like you are lifting a feather, go for the next weight, which may be twenty-five or thirty pounds.

You will quickly notice that on some exercises a beginning weight of twenty pounds is easy enough, while on other exercises that same weight is extremely difficult. For example, if you try to use twenty pounds to perform your side lateral raise you will have great difficulty. You will probably have to start with five or ten pounds for that exercise. Weight training employs different weights for different exercises, depending on the specific muscle being challenged. Smaller muscles, such as in the shoulders, require lighter weights than do larger muscles in the chest. Experimentation will quickly tell you which weights are appropriate for each exercise. As long as you can get twelve to fifteen repetitions for the first set *without too much strain and yet with some effort,* you know that the weight you are using is appropriate.

What If the Lightest Weight Is Too Heavy?

You may run into a situation where you cannot get twelve to fifteen repetitions for your first set even with the lightest weight available. Don't worry. Just do as many repetitions as possible with the lowest weight available. Eventually you will gain the strength required to complete the fifteen reps, and one day you will even increase the weight. For example, you may find that on the machine cable crossover, the first and only beginning weight is ten pounds. Perhaps you can manage only five repetitions with that weight. Fine. Just do the five, stop, do another five and stop, and do another set. Obviously you will not be able to pyramid, so do your three sets with the same weight. Later, when you can do fifteen reps easily with the ten pounds, you will be ready to pyramid your second set.

HOW TO PYRAMID YOUR WEIGHTS

As noted previously, the secret to this muscle-implant program is pyramiding. You must raise the weight for each succeeding set. Since there are three sets per exercise, you will be raising the weight twice after the initial weight. The only two body parts you will not pyramid are the abdominals and the buttocks.

When you perform your second set (beginning on your second training week), select a weight you can use to get eight to ten repetitions without lurching or misperforming the exercise. Do the ten repetitions and rest for thirty seconds. When you perform your third set (beginning on your third training week), get a higher weight, one you can use to perform six to eight repetitions without doing the exercise in a lopsided fashion.

Here is an example.

Bench Press

Set 1.	20 pounds	12–15 repetitions
Set 2.	30 pounds	8–10 repetitions
Set 3.	40 pounds	6–8 repetitions

Side Lateral Raise

Set 1.	5 pounds	12–15 repetitions
Set 2.	8 pounds	8–10 repetitions
Set 3.	12 pounds	6–8 repetitions

Remember: The rule of thumb is, if you can't get the full twelve to fifteen repetitions on the lowest weight, simply remain at the same weight (do not pyramid), and do all three sets getting as many repetitions for each set as possible. Naturally your first set should yield the most reps because you have your first energy shot for that body part.

The pyramiding system provides a natural warmup, greatest possible muscle growth, and minimum boredom.

Increasing the Weight after a Month or So

After a few weeks of working out you may find that you are having an easy time of it. You're getting your fifteen repetitions with your first set without any trouble at all. Even your second set at the higher weight is easy, and you get your ten repetitions without much of a struggle. Your third set, eight reps, also gives you little worry. When this happens, it is a sure sign that it's time to increase your weights.

In order to make more progress, to challenge the muscles to grow, you must increase the demand upon them when the work becomes too easy. This is the principle of progression, discussed earlier. You make progress by adding to the challenge when the work becomes easy.

In order to ensure the development of the shapely muscles you want under previously sagging skin, you'll have to spur yourself on by starting your first set with the next highest weight. For example, if in the bench press your first beginning weight was twenty pounds and your second and third sets were at thirty and forty, now you will begin with thirty pounds for your first set, and your second and third sets will be at forty and fifty. Now may be the time to take advantage of the leeway given you in the repetitions. You may have noticed that I allow twelve to fifteen reps for the first set, eight to ten reps for the second set, and six to eight reps for the third set. When you increase the weight, it is perfectly all right to do the lower number of repetitions if it is too difficult for you to do the full number. When you gain more strength you will be doing the full number, and then in time you'll be increasing your weights again. Roberta (a "before" and "after" in this book, see Chapter 11) started out by doing all three sets of the bench press with twenty pounds. Now her beginning weight is sixty-five pounds. She does her second set at seventy-five pounds and her last set at eighty-five pounds. I started out doing my first set at thirty pounds, but I still haven't advanced as far as Roberta. My beginning set on the bench press is sixty pounds. Barbara (also a "before" and "after" in this book) started out with a beginning weight of twenty pounds. In three months she advanced to a beginning weight of thirty-five pounds.

MUSCLE CONSCIOUSNESS

Use the anatomy pictures to locate your muscles (pages 48–49). Find your biceps, triceps, chest (pectorals), shoulders (deltoids), back (trapezius and latissimus dorsi), legs (quadriceps, hamstrings, calves), buttocks (gluteus maximus), and abdominals. Study the anatomy pictures and then look in the mirror and flex (squeeze together and tighten) each muscle separately. Remember where the muscle is so that while you are working out you can concentrate on that muscle.

Flexing during the Workout

Always flex the muscle on the contraction of each exercise. For example, on the bench press, squeeze your chest muscles together when you push the bar up. On the biceps curl, squeeze together and tighten your biceps when you curl the weight upward.

Stretching during the Workout

The action complementary to flexing is stretching. For example, on the bench press, let your chest muscles stretch out when you lower the bar to your chest. Let your biceps muscle stretch out when you lower your arm (uncurl it) on the biceps curl. It will anyway, but mentally cooperate with it. Flexing and stretching triple your progress.

A Reminder about Visualization

Don't forget to visualize the muscle growing, expanding, pumping full of blood, forming into the perfectly shaped muscle you have in mind.

Soreness: What to Expect

Even though you are only working out for about twenty minutes the first day, you will experience quite a bit of soreness the next day, especially on body parts you have particularly neglected over the years. "My back was so stiff," says Jennifer, forty-three. "It was the strangest feeling. I could hardly roll out of bed. All the rest was just minor aches."

The soreness will be greatest after the first two workouts because you are exercising different body parts on either day. After the second two workouts you will still feel sore, but to your surprise you will find that when you work the sore body part it actually feels better. "I felt much better when I left the gym the second time I worked my legs," says Marilyn, "even though it hurt a little to do the exercises with sore legs."

Working through the soreness serves as a natural message for the aching muscle to develop greater strength. Whatever you do, don't stop working out with the goal of waiting until the soreness goes away. Your muscle will just go back to sleep again. The only way to get your muscle past the point of initial soreness is train it to handle the new exercise.

Since you are adding a set for each exercise the second week, you can expect some soreness, but usually not as much as you felt the first week. On your third week you will be adding still another set, so once again there will be some soreness, but again the soreness will be noticeably less than it was in the beginning.

Soon you will feel totally comfortable lifting the weights, and the only soreness you will experience is really just a tightness that comes from pumping the weights. Other than that, the only time you might experience aches and pains will be when you raise your weights or do the "bombing" routines given in Chapter 10.

Soreness usually sets in between twelve and twenty-four hours after your workout. A hot shower or bath helps to relieve the achy feeling, but as Barbara said when I asked why she seemed so happy if she was so sore, "I love it. It makes me feel great, as if I am getting somewhere. Why, I'm using muscles I never had. I love it." I then quoted to her the "No pain, no gain" slogan, a saying that has brought comfort to aspiring athletes for many years.

You can look forward to little soreness after a month of training.

WORKOUT CLOTHING

When choosing workout clothing, the key is to suit yourself. Your personality should determine the clothes you buy. I usually wear shorts and a cutoff top with sneakers and sox. Other women in my gym wear leotards and tights. I can't stand anything restricting my legs. I like to have them free to breathe and sweat.

Whatever you do, don't just throw on old mismatched clothing, not even if you are very out of shape and don't want to spend money on clothing. You'll depress yourself if you fall into this trap. Buy colors that you like. Match your sox to your shirt or to your headband or sweats—whatever.

If you are in a gym where everyone wears sweats and you like to wear shorts, by all means do so, as long as they don't have rules regarding clothing. A gym with rules about clothing is not for me. Chances are such a gym will have lots of rules about everything, and the last thing I need when I'm trying to work out is the hindrance of rules. The philosophy of most bodybuilding gyms is live and let live. It is the fancy health spa type of gym that tends to have lots of restrictions. Be yourself in the gym. That's what counts.

WHAT ABOUT THE AEROBICS REQUIREMENT?

I suggest that you do not begin to add in your aerobic requirement until you have completed your third week of weight training. Then follow this progression to break into aerobics.

Week One of Aerobics

Select any three days as discussed before and perform five minutes of aerobics. Choose your own activity, whether it be running, jogging in place on the jogging machine, riding the stationary bicycle, or jumping rope.

Week Two of Aerobics

Add five minutes to your aerobics exercise so that you are now doing ten minutes. Do the ten minutes on each of the three aerobics days.

Week Three of Aerobics

Add five minutes to your aerobics for a total of fifteen minutes a day. Do the fifteen minutes on each of the three aerobic days.

Week Four of Aerobics

This is a special week because now you move up to your full twenty-minute aerobic requirement. Add five minutes to the fifteen you were doing last week, and you are doing twenty minutes of aerobics. If you are ambitious, at some time in the future you may go on adding minutes to your aerobic sessions.

GYM WORKOUTS VERSUS HOME WORKOUTS

There are advantages and disadvantages to both gym workouts and workouts at home. Your decision where to work out will depend upon your life-style and your psychological needs.

Advantages and Disadvantages of Home Workouts

Working out at home saves time in travel, eliminates the price of a gym membership, gives you complete privacy (you may be embarrassed to be seen in public with what you consider to be a terribly out-of-shape body), and allows you to choose your workout times more freely.

On the down side, a home workout leaves you open to interruptions such as the doorbell, the telephone, family members, and visual distractions. There are also many temptations at home that can lure you into neglecting your workout: the television, the telephone, the refrigerator, even the bed or household chores. At home you may become discouraged with no one else around to create an atmosphere of encouragement. While you may have thought to hide your body was a good idea, you might find that exposing it to others' praise and "go for it" comments would have been a better idea. Finally, since at home you have total freedom with respect to workout hours, it may be tempting to miss a workout. You may tell yourself, "I'll get up and work out from 2:00 A.M. till 3:15," and then never get up.

Yet with all things considered, if you are able to discipline yourself—to make a very specific workout schedule and stick to it—and if you are self-motivated and don't need or want anyone around and can unplug the telephone, and not answer the door, and block out all distractions, a home workout may be ideal for you.

Advantages and Disadvantages of a Gym Workout

The atmosphere of the gym provides encouragement. There is always someone around to make a comment like "You're really working hard today," or "Looking good." In addition, you can call on someone to help you if you are having trouble getting that last repetition. In the gym everyone has a common goal: to get and stay in shape, so there should be minimum distractions. Everyone should be concentrating on his or her workout.

The gym also has equipment that you could never afford to buy for the home. Some of the machines available in gyms cost thousands of dollars, and these machines often help to round out your workout and prevent the kind of boredom you might suffer from a total free weight routine at home.

The best part of the gym is the social life. You meet people with common interests, and you share ideas about that interest. I look forward to seeing my fellow gym members, even if I don't have time to chat with them. Just working alongside them makes me feel as if I am a member of a group of winners and proud to be a part of that group. Just a nod signifying "Hi" and a smile of recognition is enough to make me work out with a calm assurance. We're in this together.

The most delightful thing about gym camaraderie is the feeling of having worked up a good sweat and exchanging recognition with another gym member—he or she says, "What a workout," and you say, "I know what you mean," as you both stride out of the place armed with energy for life's demands.

There are few disadvantages to a gym, other than that it takes time to get there and you have to pay for a membership.

Choosing a Gym

There is a world of difference between a bodybuilding gym and a health spa. While some health spas will allow you enough freedom to work as you will on the equipment, many of them stress circuit training. This method of working out with weights requires you to do one set on each machine, moving quickly from one to another. Circuit training helps to tone muscle and increase aerobic capacity, but it does nothing to build the muscle that will reshape your body. If you join a gym where most people are circuit training, you will run into a problem when you want to do your three sets on a given machine. Someone will say, "Excuse me but it's my turn." He or she will not understand your explanation that you cannot give up the machine until you have performed your three sets. What is worse, even if you let someone do a set, there will be another person behind that individual demanding his or her turn next. You might have to wait until a whole line is finished.

You do not need these problems. Today there are hundreds of gyms all over that stress bodybuilding, ranging from the very plain to the somewhat luxurious.

When choosing a gym, do not be influenced by the thickness of the rugs or the presence of a swimming pool, sauna and steam bath, or juice bar. The main thing to keep in mind is the workout. Notice whether people are standing around waiting for machines. See if there is a lot of chatting going on on the gym floor. Ask the owner if he is familiar with split routines and pyramiding.

People waiting and chatting are a signal that this is not a serious bodybuilding gym. You might feel out of place here. Also, if the owner knows nothing about split routines or pyramiding, chances are he is going to be unsympathetic to your program. He may try to persuade you to do something less taxing and less rewarding. Perhaps he is more interested in your membership fee than in your progress.

If there is no available gym with the perfect atmosphere, chances are you can join a less perfect gym and simply work around the obstacles. I did for a while when I was a member of a well-known name gym. Fortunately, now I have joined a simple bodybuilding gym where the owner is a former champion bodybuilder and where the members are all busy with perfecting their bodies.

Home Gym Equipment

If you choose to set up a home gym, you will need the following equipment:

- An exercise bench that adjusts to both flat and incline positions
- A padded mat about six feet by three feet or larger
- A set of dumbbells (two of each): Five, eight, ten, twelve, fifteen, twenty, and twenty-five pounds
- A barbell set: one twenty-pound bar and assorted weights
- A bench press station to fit over the exercise bench
- Ankle weights with slots for added weights up to ten pounds

Home gym equipment can be expensive if you go for the best in quality. Plastic sand-filled weights are least expensive but also least durable. On the other hand, gold-plated dumbbells are very expensive. There is a happy medium somewhere between. Consult sporting goods stores and major department store catalogs. Shop around for the deal that suits your budget.

You can purchase your weights through *Muscle and Fitness* or *Flex* magazines. They always have advertisements describing weight sets and other workout equipment. You can go to a major department store such as Sears Roebuck or to a sporting goods store such as Herman's. A relatively new company, Triangle Health and Fitness Systems, produces attractive, moderately priced weights. (They can be reached at 1-800-446-4111.) You may also want to go to a hardcore gym equipment store like Dan Lurie's, located in Springfield Gardens, Queens, New York. (You can also call them for a catalog and order by phone: 718-978-4200.)

Another possibility is to keep your eye open for ads in the commercial section of your newspaper. Many times someone is selling a gym set at a very low price. You can also go to the local gym and ask where they suggest you buy your equipment. If you are starting from scratch, you will probably end up spending about three hundred dollars for your equipment at retail.

Once you have made your decision where to work out, follow the routines given for your workout situation. Chapter 7 describes the gym workout, and Chapter 8 describes the home workout. Carry this book to the gym or keep it in your home workout area until you are completely familiar with your routine. This may take about a month.

---

1. For more on stretching and stretch exercises, refer to Ardy Friedberg, *Reach for It* (New York: Simon and Schuster, 1983).

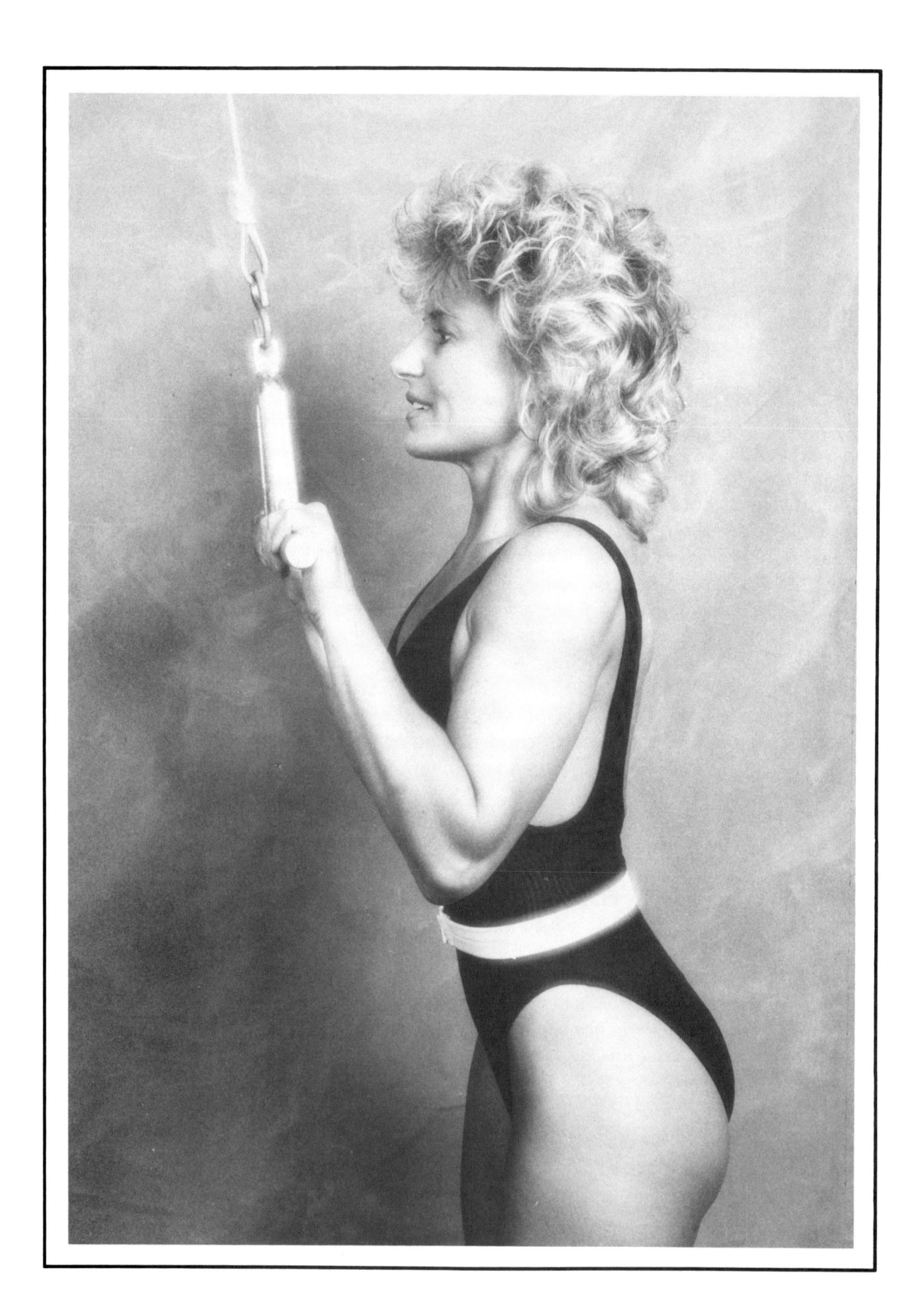

THE GYM WORKOUT

CHAPTER 7

Your gym workout will generally consist of four exercises per body part, three sets per exercise. You will be doing three times four or twelve sets per body part. On training days One and Three you will be doing chest, shoulders, back, abdominals, and buttocks. On training days Two and Four you will be doing biceps, triceps, legs, abdominals, and buttocks.

Review the bodybuilding terms at the beginning of Chapter 5 before you start. Also remember to rest as little as possible between sets. As you get used to the exercises and you develop your aerobics to the three twenty-minute sessions, you will find that your rest periods shorten from around forty-five seconds to perhaps fifteen seconds between sets.

When exercising, be alert to the tendency to hold your breath. Whenever you catch yourself doing that, force yourself to inhale on the stretching part of the exercise and exhale on the flexing (squeezing, pushing) part of the exercise. The exhaled breath will add strength to the harder, flexing part of the exercise. I don't want you to become self-conscious about your breathing, however. After a while you will be breathing naturally, and that is the best way. Some women breathe naturally from the beginning and need not concern themselves with the issue at all. Concentrate on your inhaling and exhaling only if you tend to hold your breath.

Remember to concentrate on the body part you are working. Always visualize that muscle growing and taking shape. Flex and stretch. Read the instructions and look at the pictures. Pay special attention to the "alerts" and the "nevers."

Don't forget. You begin to pyramid on Week Two and you'll be doing a full program by Week Three (see pages 71–73).

There is nothing sacred about the order of the exercises. If after a while you want to work your shoulders first and then your chest and back, fine. Just be sure to do *all* the shoulder exercises before advancing to the next body part. Often, women will do a weak body part first. They want to give it their first shot of energy.

There is also nothing sacred about the order of the particular exercises for each body part. For example, I tell you to do the bench press first and then incline flyes and next cross bench pullovers and finally cable crossovers for your chest routine. After a while you may find that you prefer to do the cable crossovers first and then the incline flyes, etc. That is fine with me—as long as you do all of your chest exercises together. *Never* mix different body part exercises together.

I advise you to follow the workout here exactly as given—in the order of presentation—until you are secure with it. I selected the order here because it is comfortable and it seems to work well for many women. Following it exactly for about three months is a good idea. Then you can go to town and move things around, as long as you know what you are doing (and believe me, by then you will).

Your beginning weight will be the lightest weight you can use and still get twelve to fifteen repetitions. If the gym has no weight light enough to get twelve to fifteen reps, just take the lightest weight they have and get in as many reps as you can (see page 74).

Right now all of this may seem so complicated that you are wondering if you can ever do it. But in about three weeks you'll think back and wonder, "What was the big deal." You'll feel like a pro. The only way to find this out is to start doing it. Plunge in and plow your way through the initial confusion. The reward will be yours very soon.

Okay, go for it. Wait until they see you in three months!

THE GYM WORKOUT 87

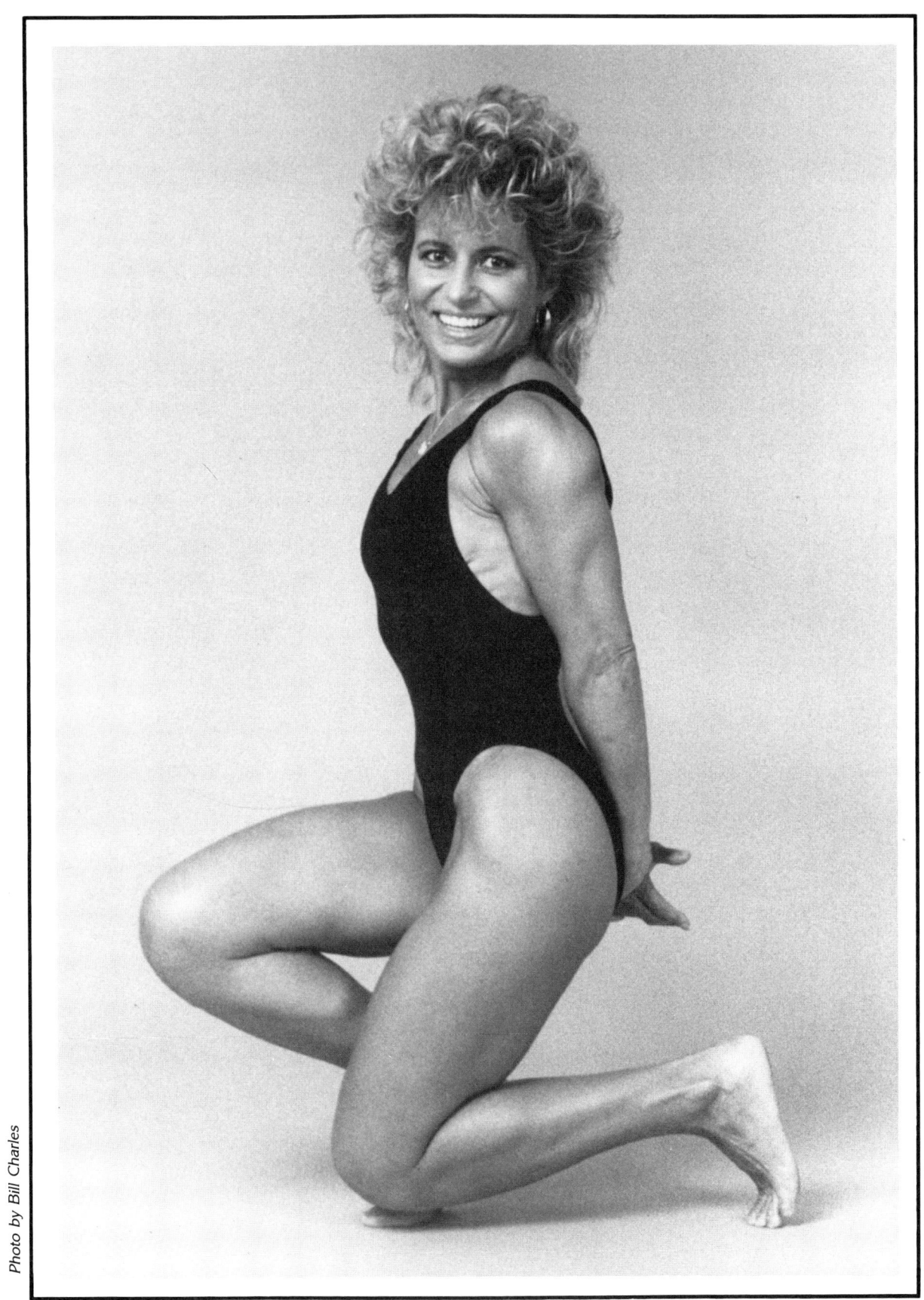

Photo by Bill Charles

CHEST ROUTINE

DAYS ONE AND THREE

Bench Press—Chest Exercise #1

This is the most basic chest (pectoral) exercise. It develops the full pectoral area and places a firm muscle under your breasts, helping to lift them and to give a look of "cleavage."

POSITIONING
- Lie on a flat exercise bench under the machine or free weight press.
- With your back flat on the bench, grip the barbell or bar with your hands about four inches wider apart than shoulder width.
- Your palms should face upward.

EXERCISE
- Lift the barbell or bar to starting position, which is straight up at arm's length.
- Slowly lower the bar until it touches your chest at the lower edge of your pectoral muscle. Stretch your chest as you do this.
- Slowly raise the bar to starting position and flex (squeeze together) your chest as you do this. Repeat the movement until you have performed the correct number of repetitions for your set.

ALERT
- Control the barbell or bar at all times, and remember to stretch and flex. Picture your muscles growing and taking shape.

"NEVERS"
- Never lopsidedly jerk the bar or barbell up using more force with one hand than the other.
- Never let the barbell almost drop onto your chest. Control the bar or barbell at all times and concentrate.

THE GYM WORKOUT **89**

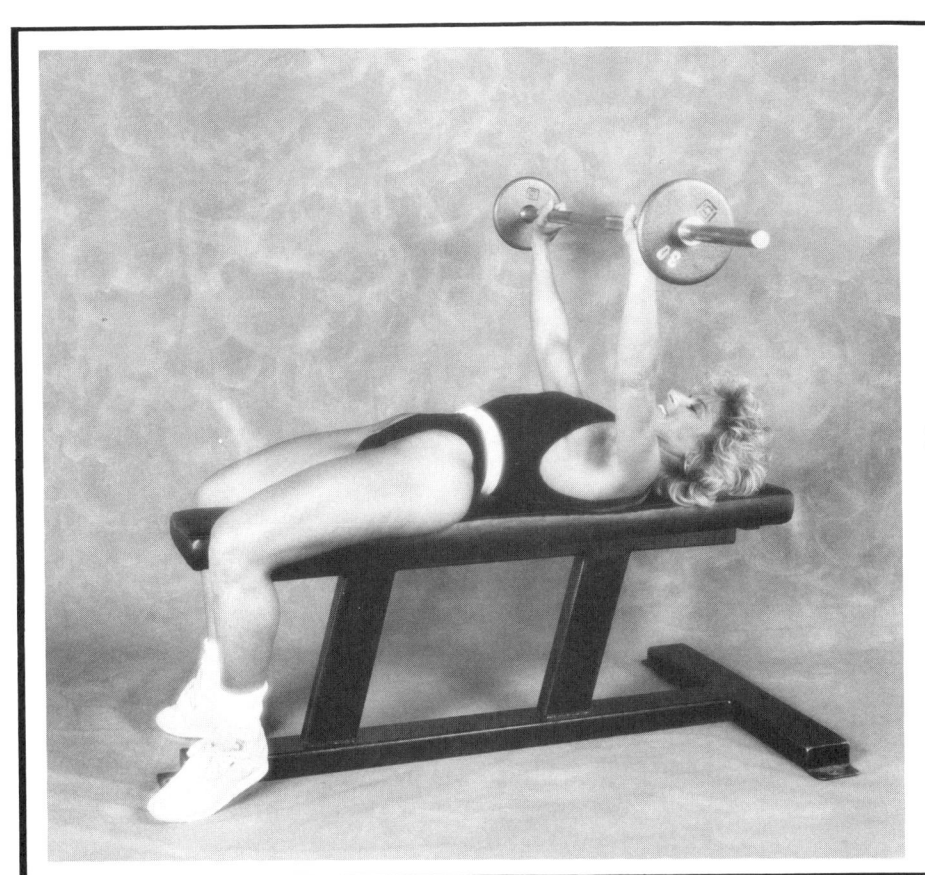

Start

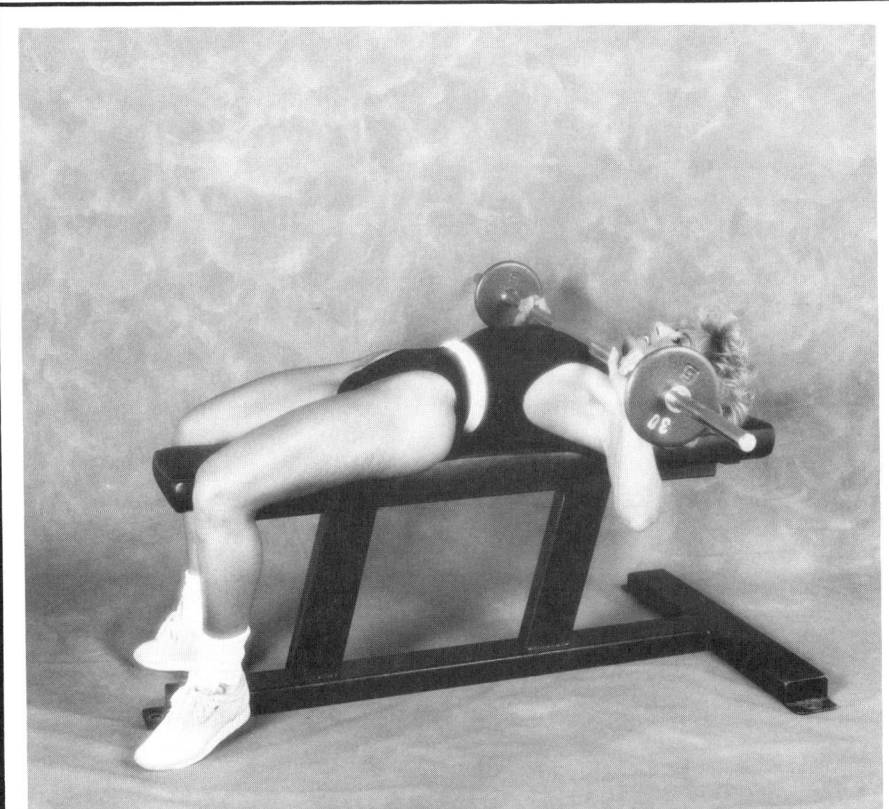

Finish

Incline Flye—Chest Exercise #2

The incline flye develops the pectoral (breast) area and slightly stresses the front deltoid (shoulder) muscle. Because the exercise is performed on an incline, the upper chest muscles are especially stressed.

POSITIONING

- Lie on an incline bench with one dumbbell in each hand.
- Extend your arms over your head so that the dumbbells are just above your shoulder joints at full arm's length.
- Keep your palms facing inward at all times.

EXERCISE

- Begin with dumbbells touching each other and slowly move them outward and downward in a semicircle on each side, moving them outward until you feel a full stretch in your chest area.
- Return to starting position, tracing the same arc pattern, and flex (squeeze together) your chest (pectoral) muscles.
- Repeat the movement until you have performed the correct number of repetitions for your set.

ALERT

- As you are moving the dumbbells to the outer position, expand your chest and stretch it as much as possible. When returning to starting position, flex (squeeze) your pectorals as much as possible.

"NEVERS"

- Never raise yourself off the bench by arching your back when performing the movement in an effort to make it "easy." If you find that you are unable to resist doing this, your weight is too heavy. Lighten it and do the exercise in strict form. Your back must remain flat on the bench at all times. Concentrate and maintain control of the weights throughout the set.

THE GYM WORKOUT **91**

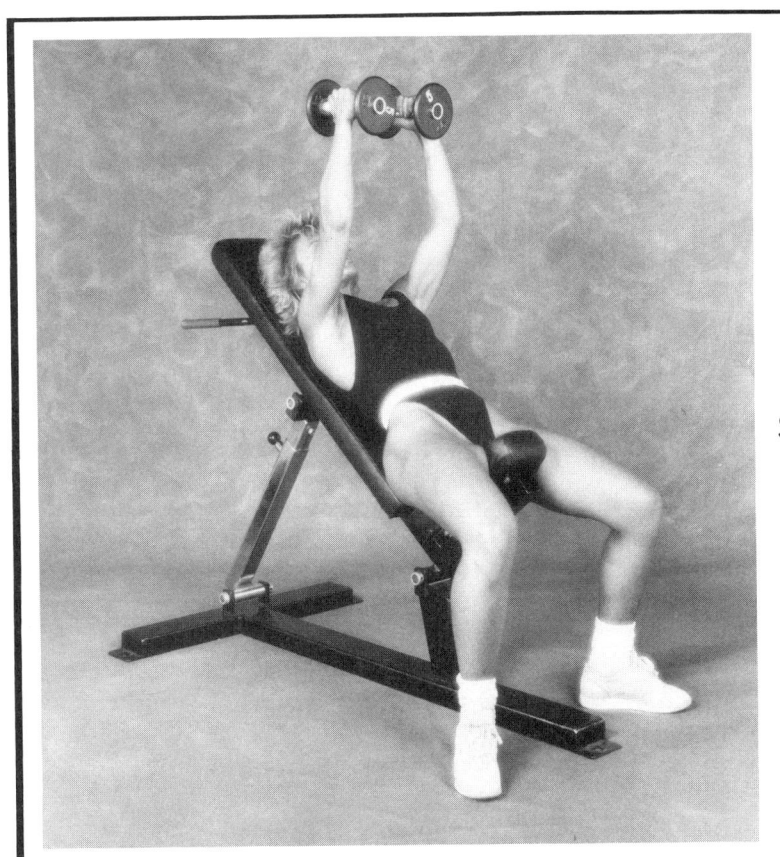

Start

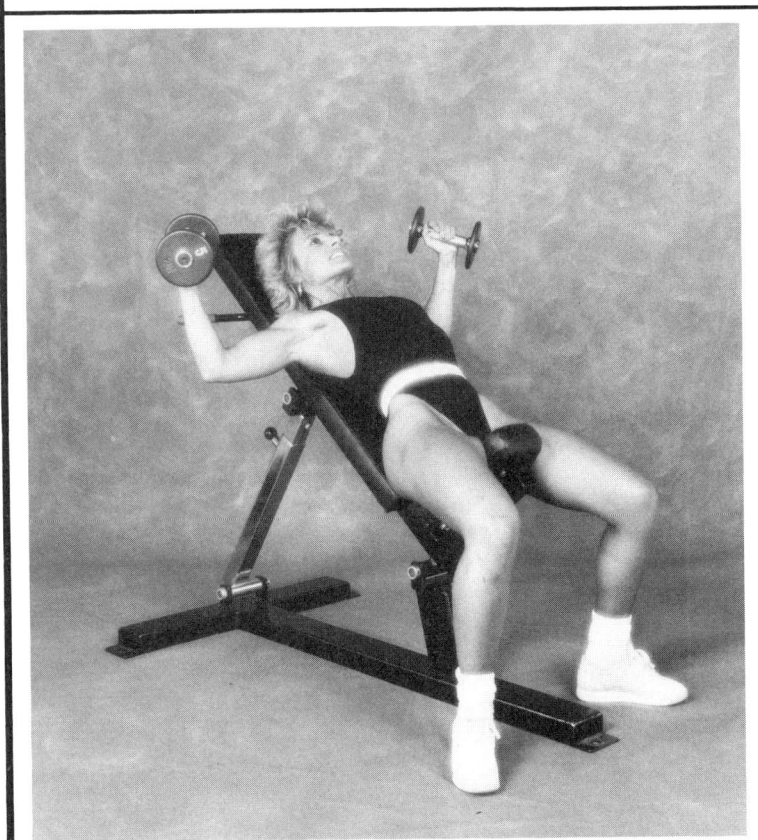

Finish

Cross Bench Pullover—Chest Exercise #3

The entire pectoral area is developed by this exercise. It helps to give the breasts an uplifted, fuller look because it places firm muscle under the fatty tissue of the breast. Some stress is placed on the side and back muscles (serratus and latissimus dorsi).

POSITIONING

- Hold a single dumbbell with both hands against the inside plate so that your thumbs are touching.
- Lean over a curved exercise bench (or a flat bench if no curved bench is available) so that your shoulders touch the highest point of the curve (or the edge of the flat bench).
- Extend your arms upward, holding the dumbbell two inches above your forehead. Keep your feet slightly apart and your knees bent.

EXERCISE

- Slowly lower the dumbbell over the bench, over your head—the dumbbell will be traveling behind you—and let it travel as low as possible until you feel a complete stretch in your chest (pectoral) area. The dumbbell will be moving in a vertical semicircle directly behind your head.
- Raise the dumbbell to start position and flex (squeeze) your pectoral muscles. Repeat the movement until you have performed the correct number of repetitions for your set.

ALERT

- If you are using a rounded bench, you will be placing your feet astride the bench and your back along the rounded part of the bench. The actual pullover will be done over the hump of the bench.

"NEVERS"

- Never let the dumbbell almost drop to its low position in an effort to avoid work. Control the dumbbell at all times as you *slowly* lower it.
- Never wildly lurch the dumbbell up to starting position in an attempt to get the exercise over with quickly. Concentrate and control the weight. Be careful to avoid hitting yourself with the dumbbell.
- Never let your mind wander.
- Never hold your breath for a few repetitions in terror of the weight. Breathe naturally. There's nothing to be afraid of. You are controlling the weight.

THE GYM WORKOUT 93

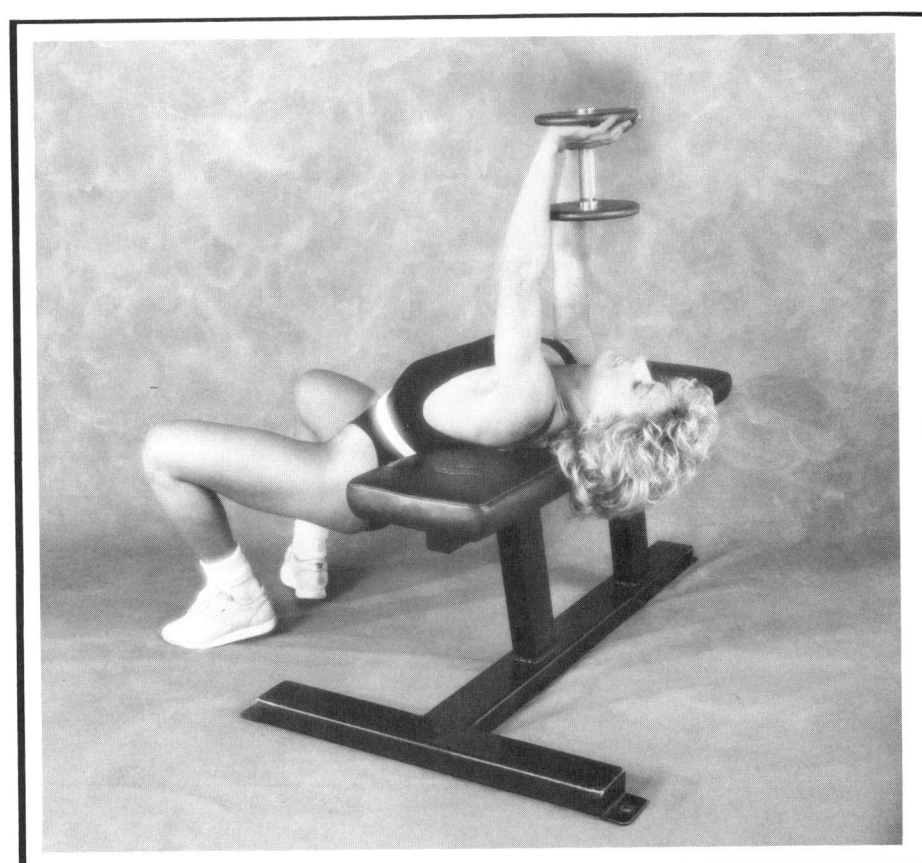

Start

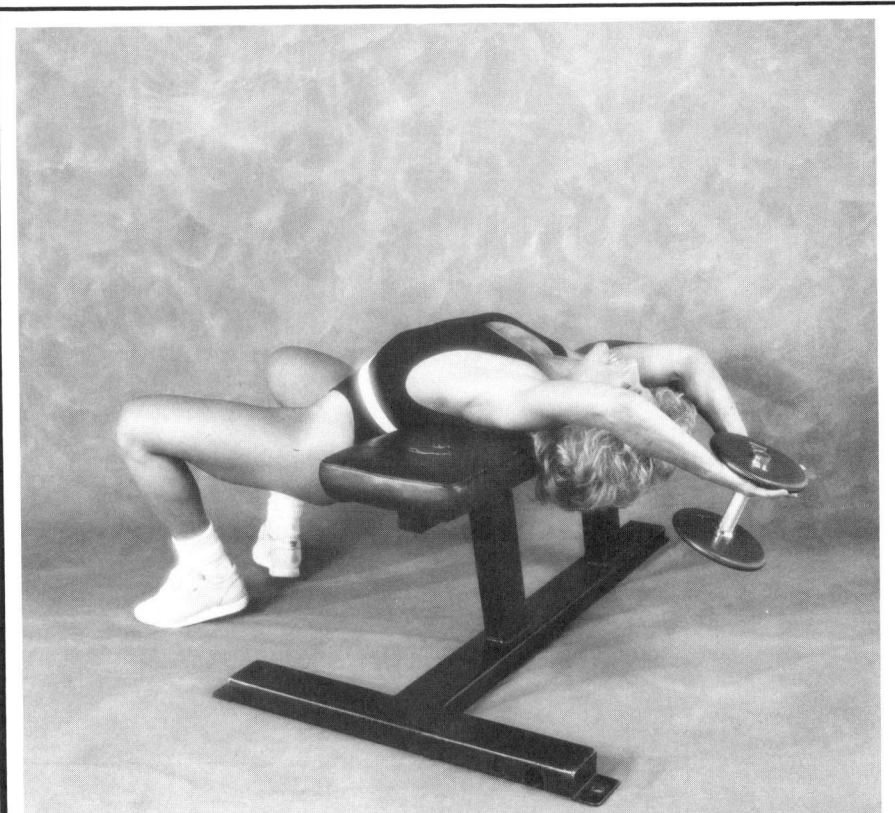

Finish

Cable Crossover— Chest Exercise #4

The inner and lower areas of the pectoral muscles are developed by this exercise. It is especially useful as a remedy for "sagging" or "drooping" breasts.

POSITIONING

- Grasp one handle of the crossover pulley machine in each hand and position yourself in the middle of the workout area, feet shoulder width apart.
- Keep your arms at a 45° upward angle, slightly bent, with hands facing downward.
- Bend forward about 15° and take a firm foot position.

EXERCISE

- Slowly pull both handles downward in an arc while flexing the pectoral (chest) muscles until the handles cross each other at the center of your body, wrist over wrist, wrists touching.
- Hold that position for one second and slowly return to starting position, being careful to control the weights at all times. Repeat the movement until you have completed the correct number of repetitions for your set.

ALERT

- This exercise can be performed one arm at a time. This allows for greater concentration and avoids "favoring" one side of the chest over the other.

"NEVERS"

- Never jerk the weight downward.
- Never let the weight pull your arms upward to starting position. Always maintain full control and fluid movement.

THE GYM WORKOUT 95

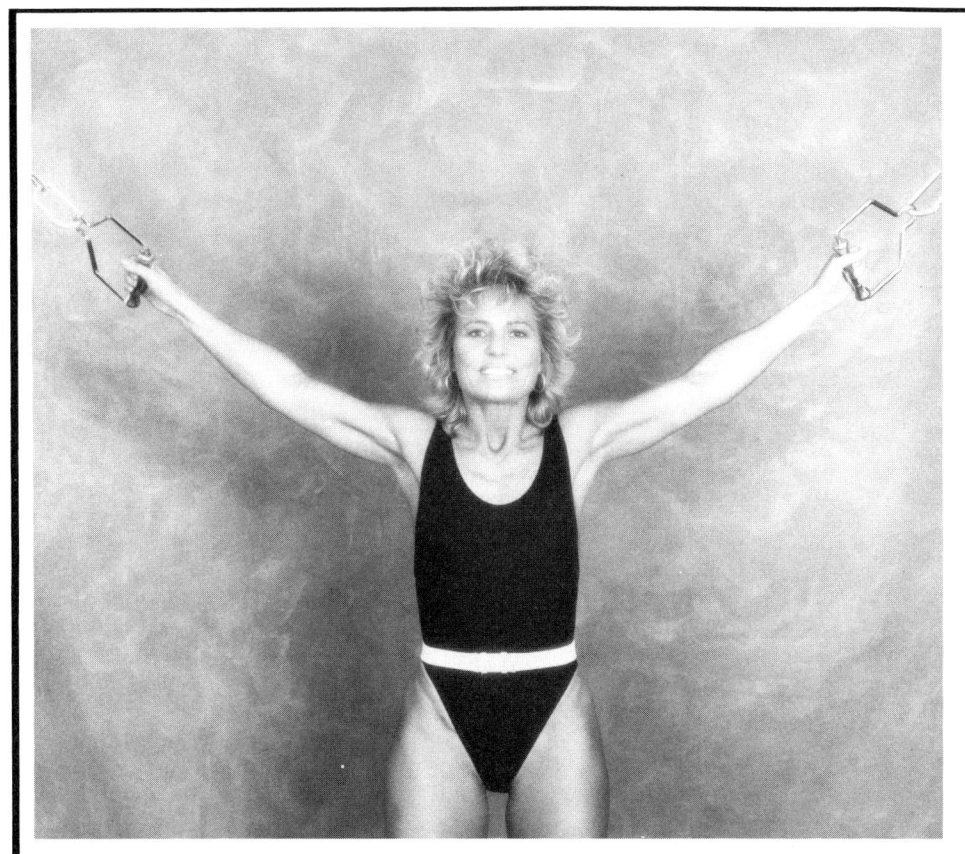

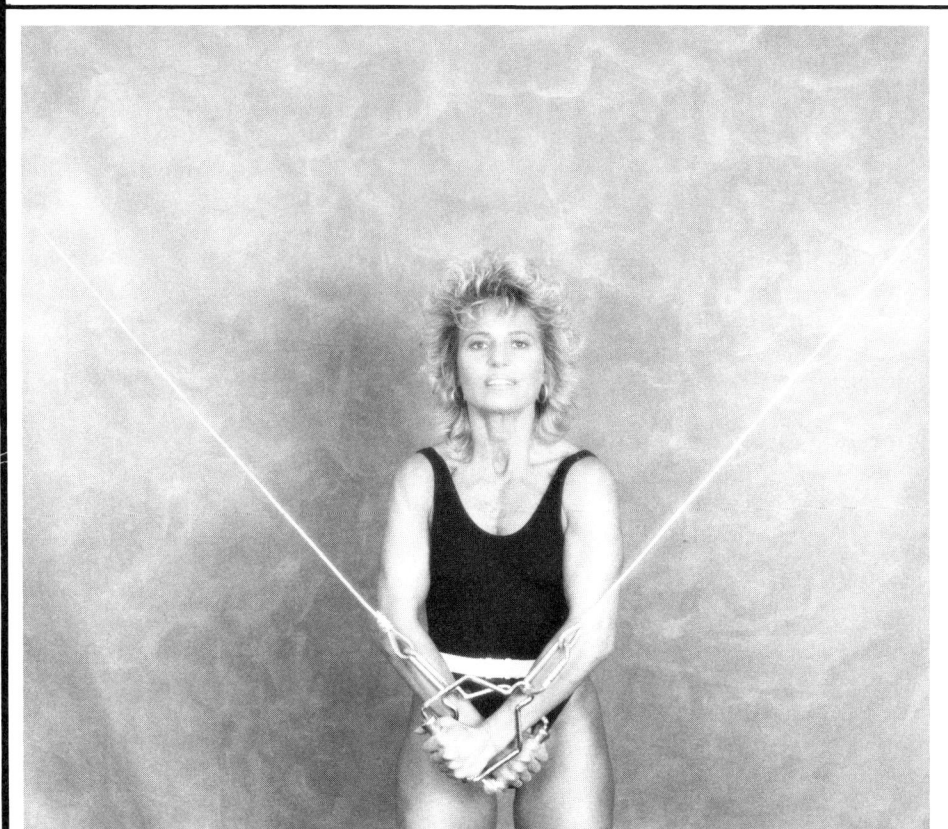

Start

Finish

SHOULDER ROUTINE

Side Lateral Raise—Shoulder Exercise #1

The front and side deltoid (shoulder) muscles will be developed by this exercise. You will see pretty lines defining your shoulder muscles in less than three months. The exercise also helps to develop the trapezius (traps), giving an esthetic look to your neck and shoulder area (see anatomy picture).

POSITIONING

- Hold one dumbbell in each hand in front of you and touch the dumbbells to each other at the center of your body.
- Lean slightly forward and bend your elbows slightly, holding your elbows about waist height.

EXERCISE

- Raise the dumbbells outward, away from your sides, slowly while flexing (squeezing together) your shoulder muscles, describing a semicircle on each side until you reach shoulder height on each side.
- Return to starting position, continuing to flex your shoulders and completely controlling the weights. Repeat the movement until you have performed the correct number of repetitions for your set.

ALERT

- By raising the dumbbells higher than shoulder height (to ear level), you will develop the trapezius muscles to a greater extent and lessen some shoulder development. If your traps really need work you should go to ear height.

"NEVERS"

- Never swing the weights up and then merely drop them down to starting position. If you cannot control the weights, use lower weights.

THE GYM WORKOUT 97

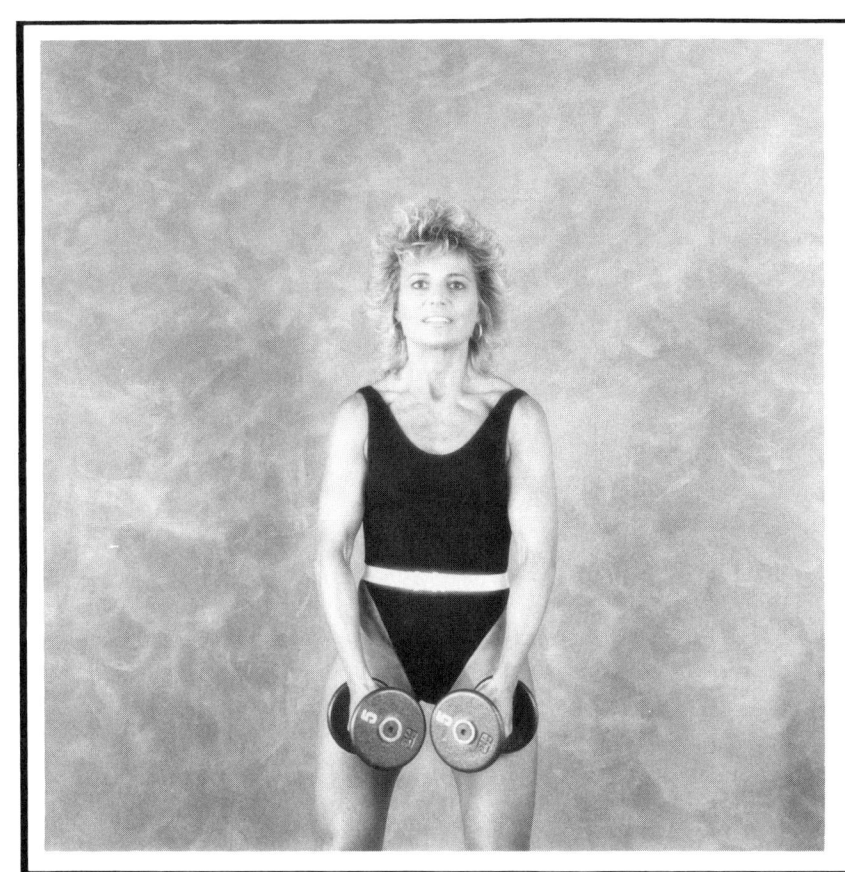

Start

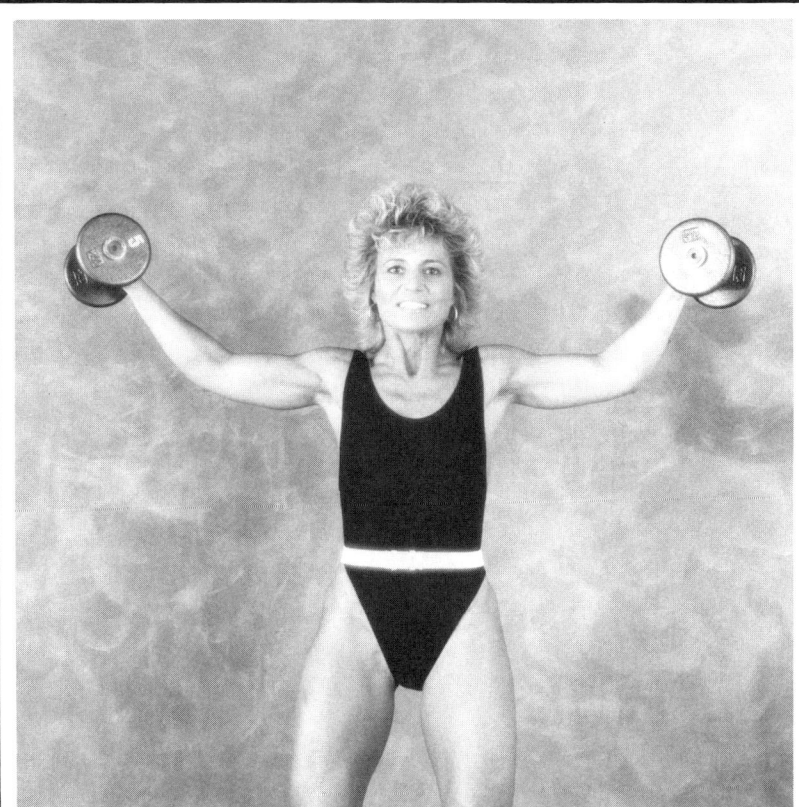

Finish

Front Lateral Raise—Shoulder Exercise #2

The front deltoid (shoulder) muscles are developed by this exercise. You will see pretty lines of definition in your front shoulder area in less than three months.

POSITIONING

- Stand with feet shoulder width apart with one dumbbell in each hand, arms straight down in front of your thighs.
- Flex your shoulders and, holding the dumbbells with palms facing your body, lean very slightly forward at the waist.

EXERCISE

- Maintaining full control, raise your right arm in front of your body to shoulder height, and while you are slowly returning to starting position, raise your left arm to shoulder height. Keep your shoulders flexed throughout the exercise.
- While you are returning your left arm to starting position, raise your right arm to shoulder height, and alternate until you have completed the correct number of repetitions for your set. Each arm should receive the correct number of repetitions for your set.

ALERT

- You may use a barbell instead of dumbbells and work both shoulders at the same time. You may want to do this once in a while to prevent boredom.
- You may use the dumbbells in unison, raising and lowering both at the same time for variety.

"NEVERS"

- Never allow your elbows to bend while performing the movement.
- Never swing your arm upward in an attempt to gain momentum and make the work easier. Control the weight at all times.

THE GYM WORKOUT **99**

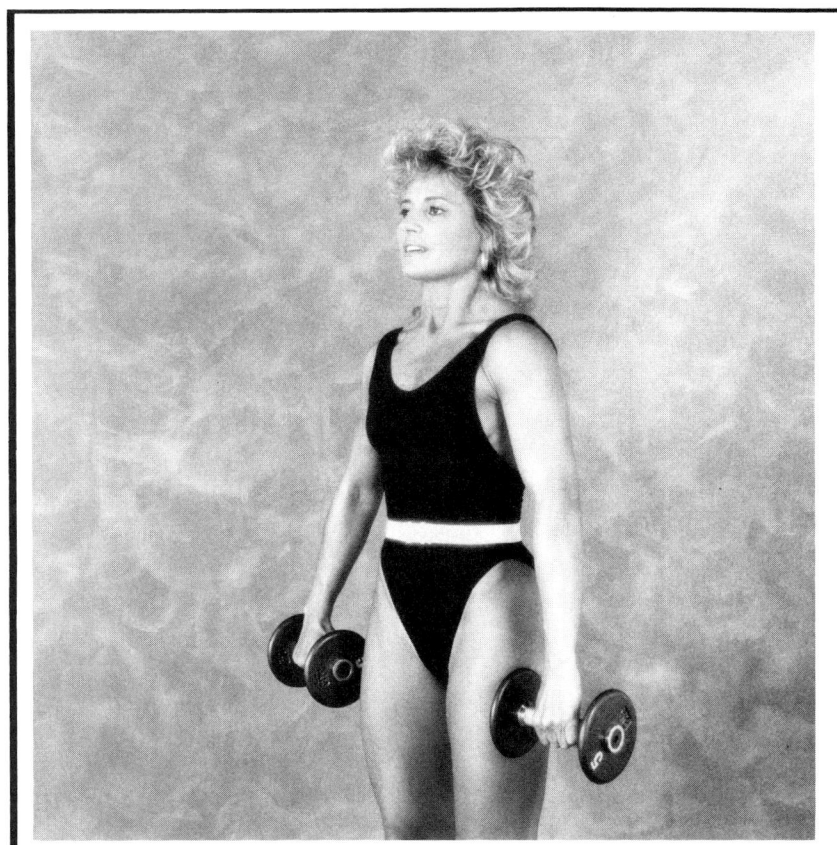

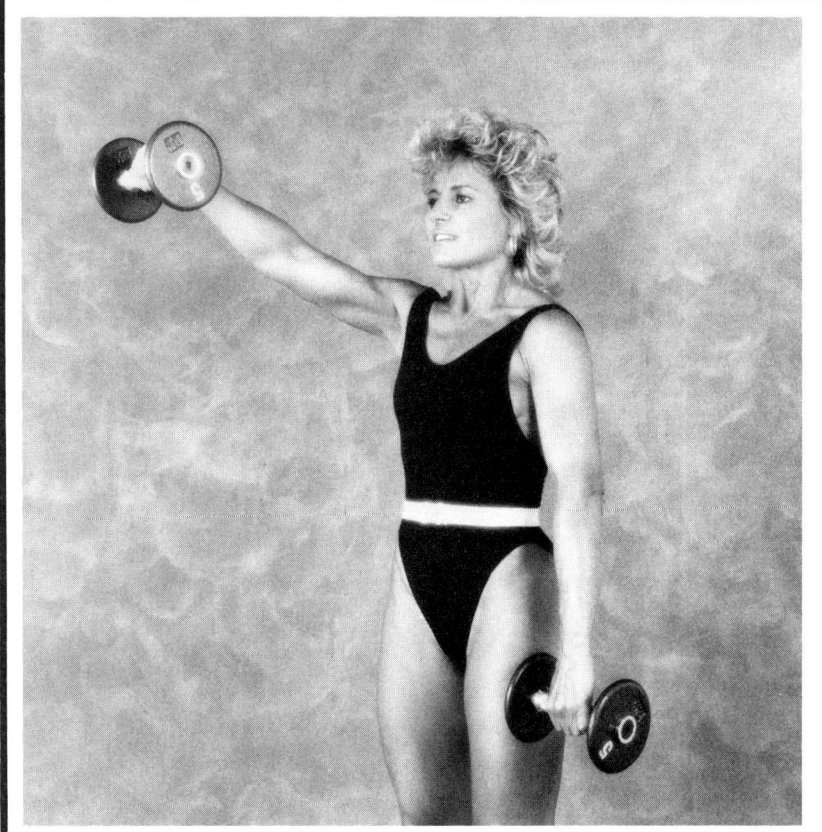

Start

Finish

Military Press behind the Neck— Shoulder Exercise #3

The front deltoids (shoulder) muscles are developed by this exercise, causing lines of definition to appear in your front shoulder area. The triceps are also slightly stressed by this movement. In addition, the trapezius muscles are developed by this movement, which is necessary to give you that symmetrical "finished" look and to avoid the "pencil neck" look.

POSITIONING

- Grip a barbell with both hands held shoulder width apart, and stand with your feet in a comfortable position (slightly less than shoulder width apart). Be sure that your palms are facing away from you.
- Place the barbell on your shoulders, resting it on your trapezius muscles. Bend your knees very slightly.

EXERCISE

- Push the barbell straight up until your arms are fully extended above your shoulders and then slowly return to starting position, flexing your shoulders as much as possible during the movement. Complete this movement until you have performed the correct number of repetitions for your set.

ALERT

- You may do an alternate military press to the front by holding the barbell in front of you, resting it on your upper chest.
- You may do back or front military presses either sitting or standing.

"NEVERS"

- Never lose control of the barbell. Make sure it is balanced on your shoulders before starting the exercise.
- Never jerk the barbell up.
- Never let the barbell simply drop to your shoulders because you are tired. Concentrate, and control the weight at all times. Make up your mind to complete the set before resting.

THE GYM WORKOUT **101**

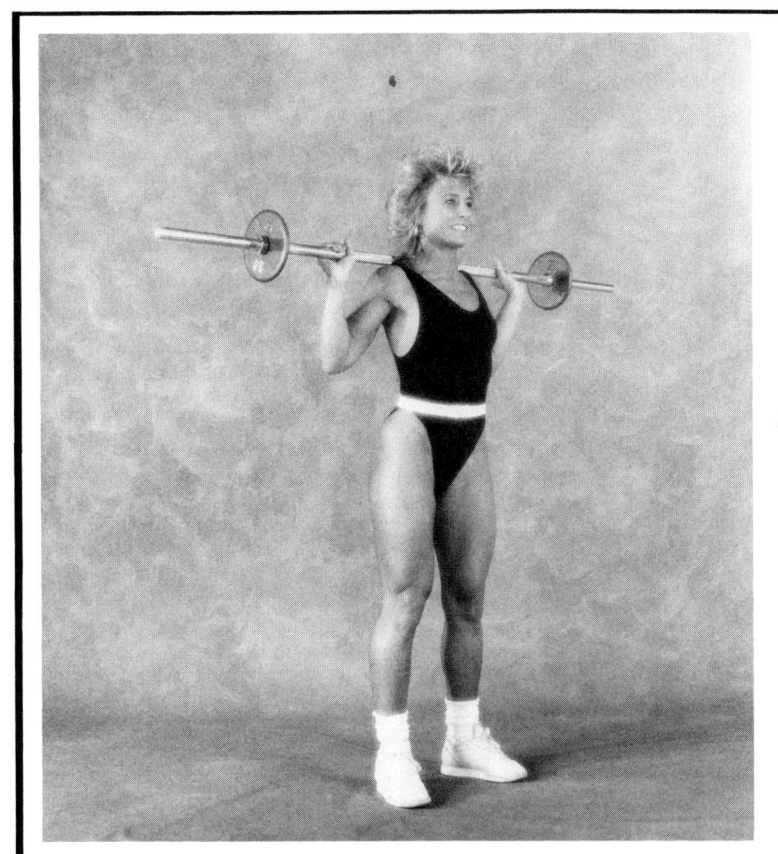

Start

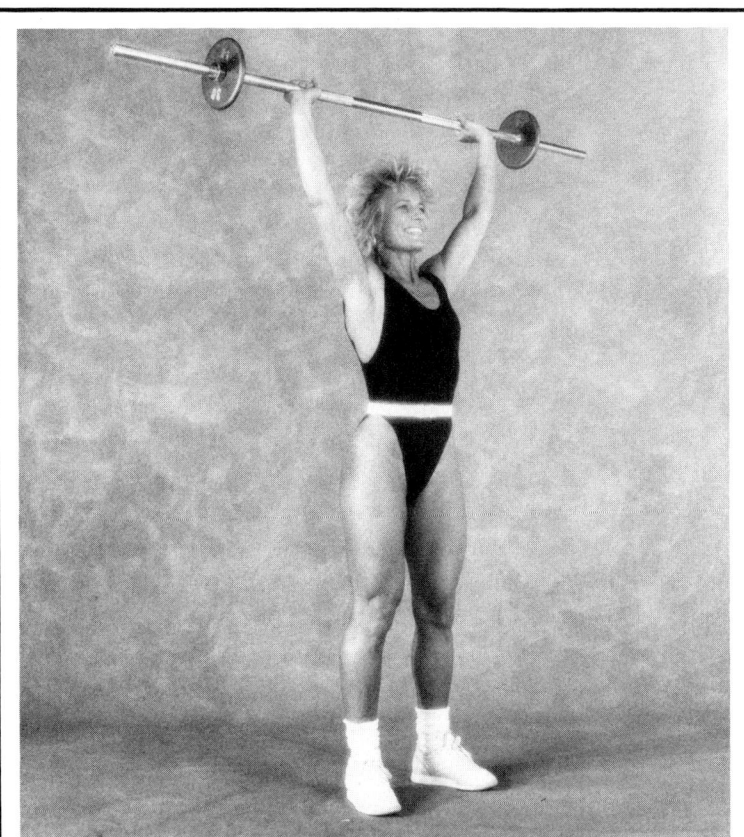

Finish

Upright Row—Shoulder Exercise #4

The entire deltoid (shoulder) area and the trapezius muscles (connecting the shoulder and the neck) are developed by this exercise.

POSITIONING

- Grasp a barbell with hands (thumbs) about six inches apart, palms facing your body.
- Let the barbell hang down as you drop your arms down to your sides. The barbell should be leaning against your upper thighs.

EXERCISE

- Pull the barbell slowly to your chin, keeping your elbows high. Be careful to stand straight. Avoid the temptation to lean forward or to bend your knees.
- When the barbell nearly touches your chin, flex your shoulder muscles and slowly return to starting position. Repeat the movement until you have performed the correct number of repetitions for your set.

ALERT

- You may alter your grip every week or so. You can grip the barbell anywhere from five to ten inches apart (distance from thumb to thumb).

"NEVERS"

- Never jerk the barbell up.
- Never let the barbell just drop into starting position in an effort to avoid work. Flex. Concentrate. Control.
- Never hold your breath for a few repetitions. Relax and remember that the weight can't hurt you. You are in control.

THE GYM WORKOUT **103**

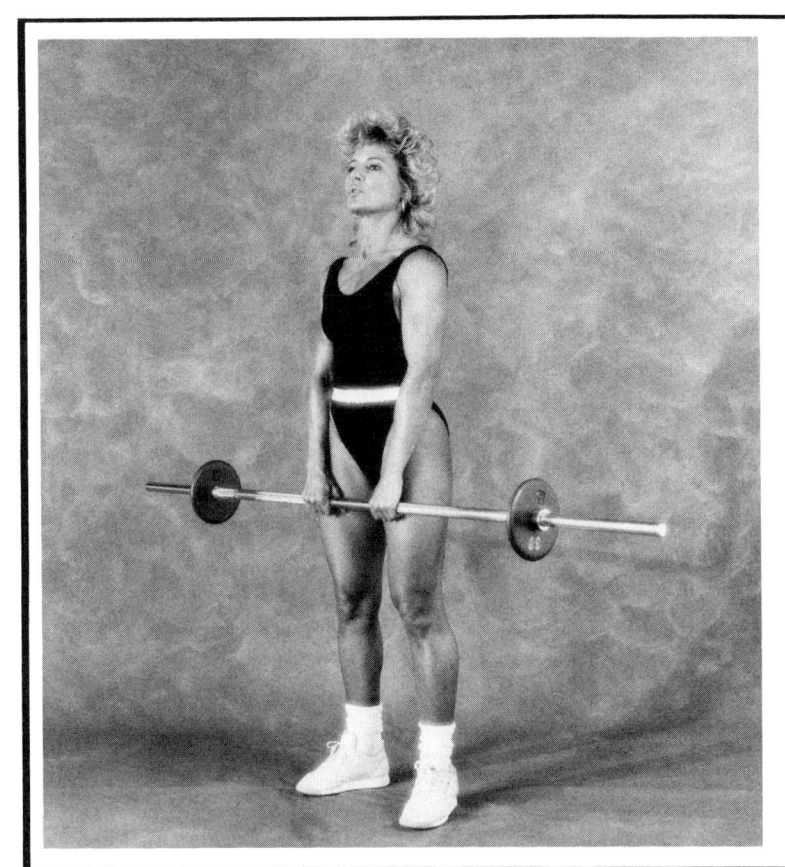

Start

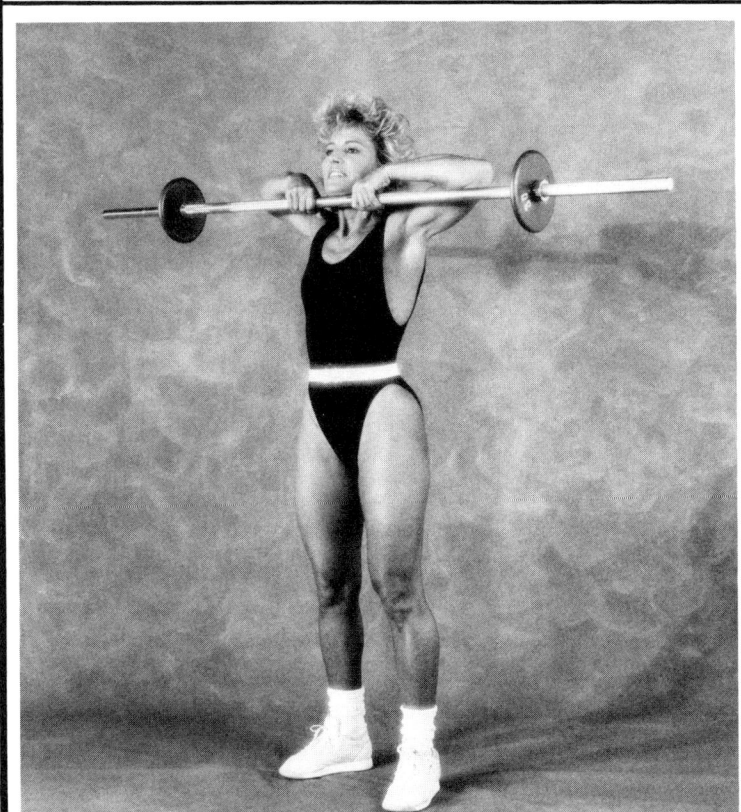

Finish

Lat Machine Pulldown to the Back— Back Exercise #1

BACK ROUTINE

The "widening" (latissimus dorsi, or "lat") muscles of your back (see the reference photos at the beginning of Chapter 5) are developed by this exercise. It can be done on any appropriate gym machine. It is described here for a free-standing lat machine.

POSITIONING

- Place yourself in position in the machine seat with your knees securely under the knee restraining bar. (You may have to adjust the seat.)
- Grip the lat machine bar with your palms forward and thumbs up, hands shoulder width apart.
- Allow your arms to be pulled until fully extended upward. You should feel the weight of the machine stretching your back.

EXERCISE

- Slowly pull the bar downward until it is touching your trapezius muscles (neck-shoulder area), making sure that you do the work with your back and not your arms. Mentally work with your back. Tell your arms not to work.
- Controlling the weight, return to starting position, making sure to get a full stretch in the back. Let the bar pull your back into a stretch. Then repeat the movement, each time letting your back do the work and letting the bar stretch your back on the return to start position.
- Repeat the movement until you have performed the correct number of repetitions for your set.

ALERT

- Control the weight at all times. Let your back do all the work.
- Squeeze your lat muscles as much as possible throughout the exercise.

"NEVERS"

- Never let yourself rise up from the seat.
- Never let the weight of the bar jerk you up into the final stretch. Control the weight and let it stretch you slowly into the start position.
- Never jerk the bar downward in an attempt to get it over with. Control the weight at all times.

THE GYM WORKOUT 105

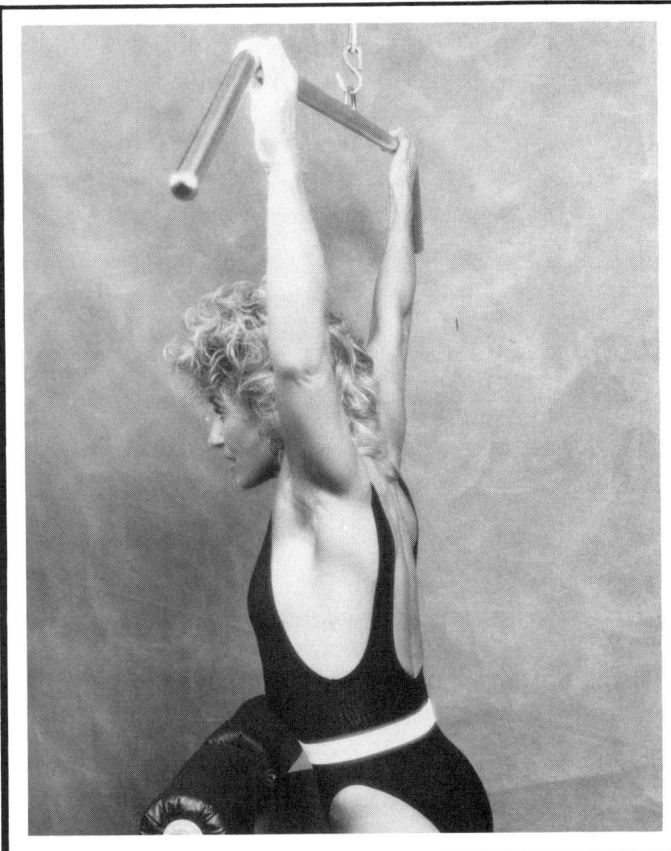

Start

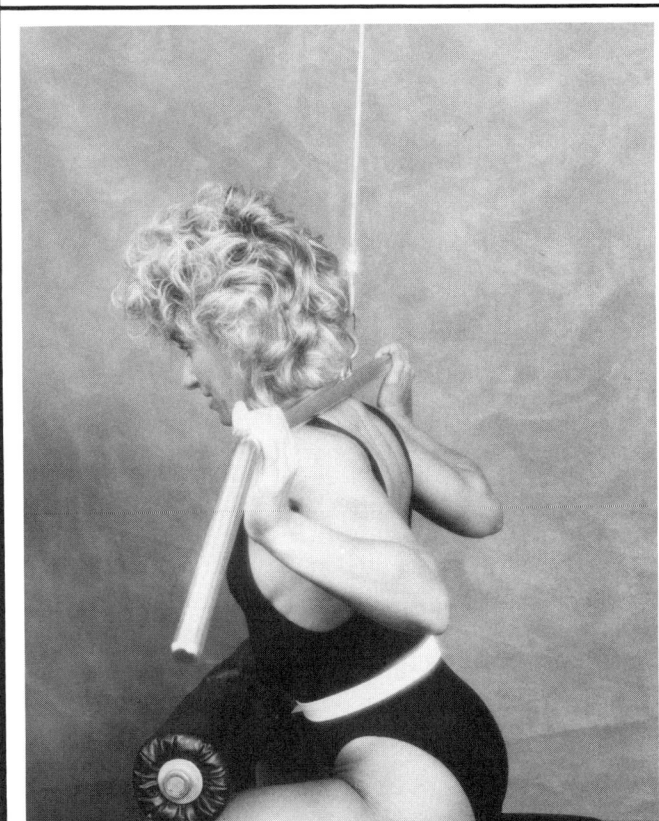

Finish

Seated Pulley Row— Back Exercise #2

The "widening" (latissimus dorsi) muscles of the upper back are developed by this exercise. It will help you to achieve the athletic V look from the back (as opposed to the misshapen look of a pear or an apple).

POSITIONING

- Sit in the seat of the pulley-row machine holding the parallel-grip handles in each hand with palms facing each other.
- Place your feet on the metal foot-rest bar. Bend your knees slightly.
- Extend your arms fully and lean forward for a full back stretch.

EXERCISE

- Pull the handles toward your chest, bending your arms and straightening your back at the same time. Your body should end up in a perpendicular position. Do not lean backward.
- Touch the handles to your upper abdomen and push your chest out, arching your back. Keep your upper arms close to your body at all times.
- Return to starting position and repeat the movement until you have performed the correct number of repetitions for your set.

ALERT

- It is a good idea to start your back routine with this exercise if your back is a little stiff. It provides a natural stretch.
- Remember to stretch as far forward as possible each time you return to starting position and to stretch your back muscles fully. Imagine the muscles expanding and taking the shape of a V. Flex (squeeze) your back muscles as you pull the handles toward your chest.

"NEVERS"

- Never let the weights pull you forward to starting position. Instead, control the weights and slowly return to start each time.
- Never let yourself fall into the trap of leaning backward in an attempt to make the exercise easier. Maintain a perpendicular position on the finish position each time. If you cannot do that, lower your weight.

THE GYM WORKOUT 107

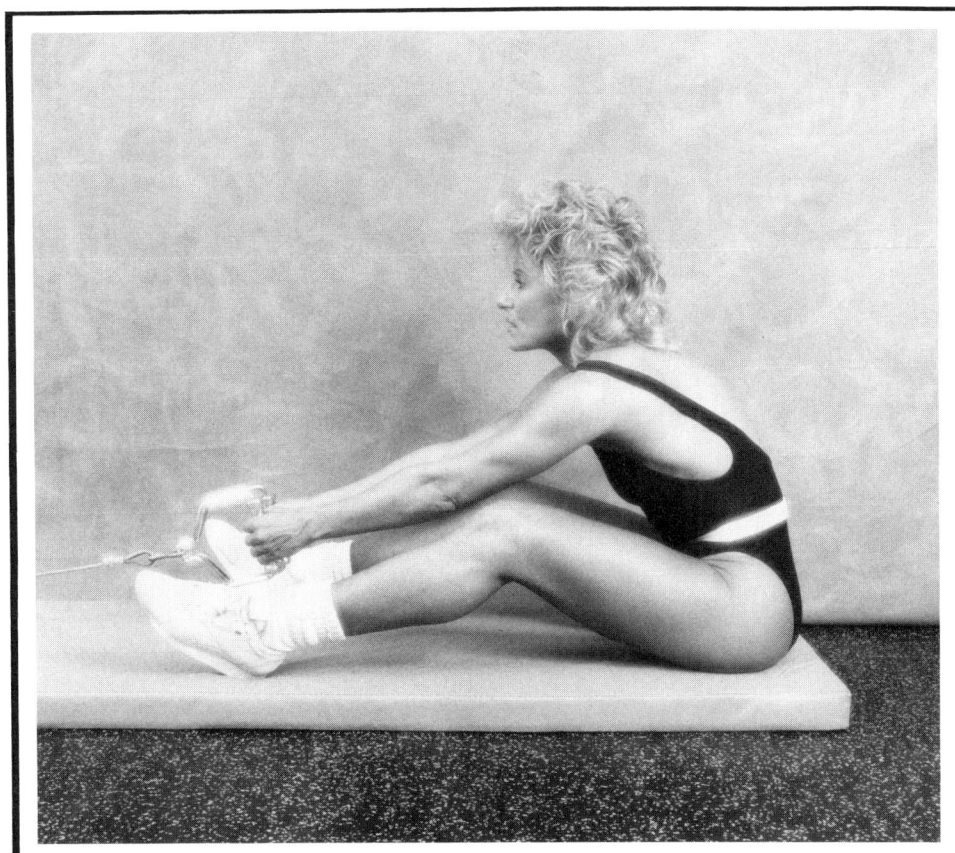

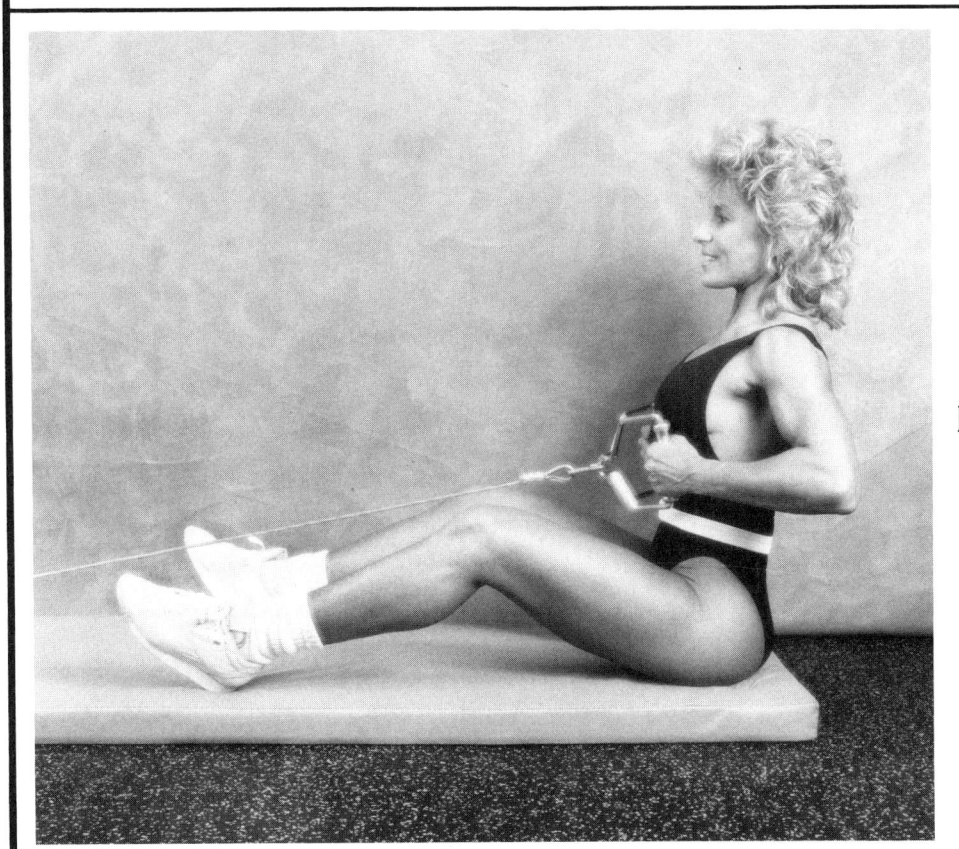

Start

Finish

One-Arm Dumbbell Bent Row— Back Exercise #3

This exercise adds thickness to the back and develops the latissimus dorsi. It also helps to create the athletic *V* look.

POSITIONING

- Kneel on a flat exercise bench with your left leg, letting your right leg extend straight to the floor.
- Holding a dumbbell in your right hand, let your right arm hang down directly in line with your shoulder joint. Let the dumbbell "stretch out" your back.

EXERCISE

- Pull the dumbbell up to your waist, at the same time slightly moving your hip to cooperate with the exercising arm. Keep your elbow close to your side.
- Maintaining control, lower the dumbbell to starting position. Be sure to feel a stretch in your back on the downward move. Repeat the movement until you have performed the correct number of repetitions for your set.
- Change to the other arm and perform the correct number of repetitions for your set. Alternate right arm and left until you have completed the correct number of sets for your routine.

ALERT

- When your arm has reached the starting position (hanging down), be sure to let the dumbbell stretch your back. Pause a split second before pulling the dumbbell to the up position.

"NEVERS"

- Never let the weight merely fall as you lower it.
- Never jerk the weight up to position. Maintain control at all times.

THE GYM WORKOUT **109**

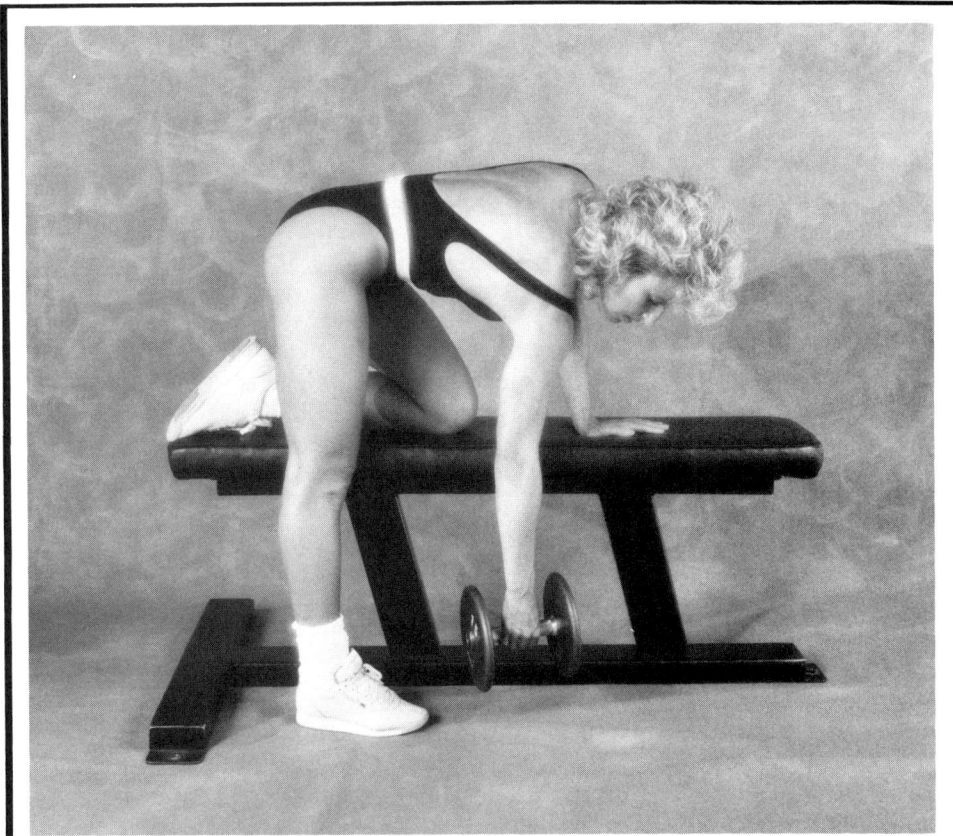

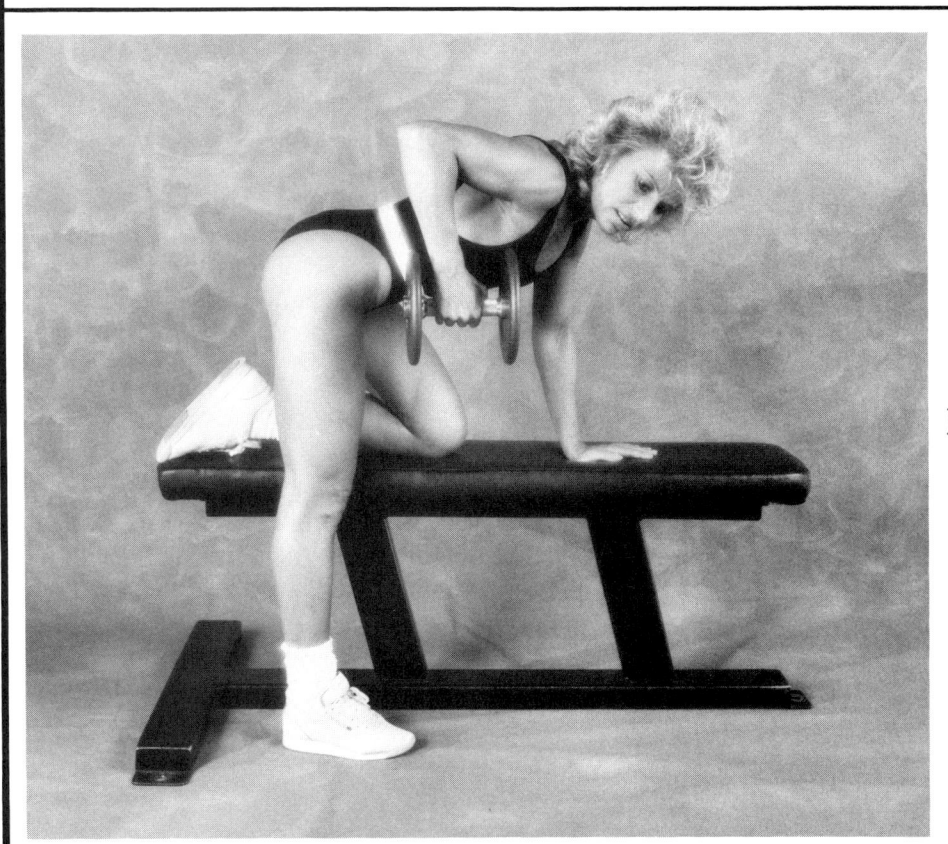

Start

Finish

Lat Machine Pulldown to the Front—Back Exercise #4

The middle and lower latissimus dorsi, or "lats," are developed by this exercise. It can be done on any appropriate gym machine. If a looped bar is available, use that. Otherwise use the regular lat machine bar. This exercise is performed in similar fashion to the lat pulldown to the back, only this time you are bringing the bar down to your chest.

POSITIONING

- Place yourself in position in the machine seat with your knees securely under the knee-restraining bar. You may have to adjust the seat. If there is no restraining bar, simply hold your body from rising by concentration.
- Grip the lat machine bar by the looped handles, palms facing your head. If you are using a regular lat machine bar, grip the bar about four inches wider than shoulder width on each side.
- Allow the weight to pull you up into a stretch. Your arms should be fully extended upward.

EXERCISE

- Slowly pull the bar downward until it is touching your upper chest. Be sure to do the work with your lat muscles and not with your arms. Flex (squeeze) your back muscles in the down position. Return to start and repeat the movement until you have performed the correct number of repetitions for your set.

ALERT

- Control the weight at all times, and remember to let the weight stretch your back on the start movement. You may even pause for a split second to allow your lats to be stretched and expanded.
- Be sure that your back does the work, not your arms.

"NEVERS"

- Never let the bar pull your body off the seat in a jerky fashion. Ground your body to the seat mentally.
- Never plunge the weight downward in an effort to finish the movement quickly. Instead, slowly and in a controlled fashion guide the weight down into the finish position.

Turn to pages 138–153 and do your Abdominal and Buttocks Routines.

THE GYM WORKOUT **111**

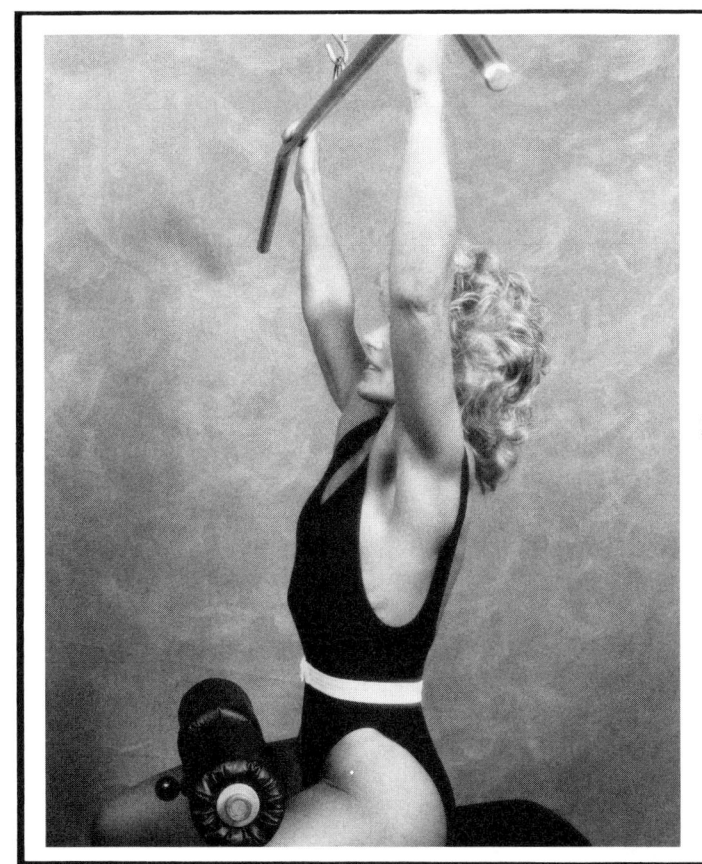

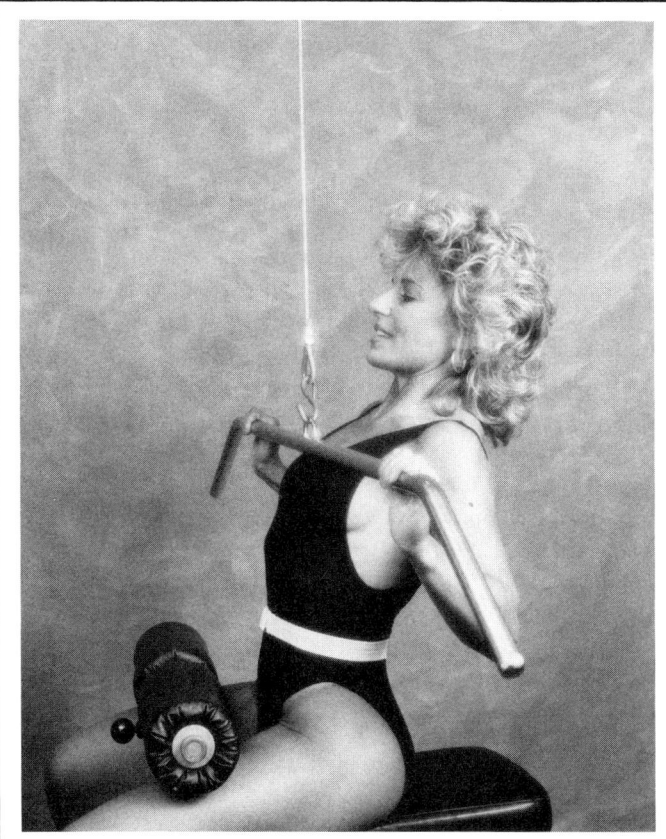

Start

Finish

BICEPS ROUTINE

DAYS TWO AND FOUR

Standing Barbell Curl—Biceps Exercise #1

The entire biceps area of the arm is developed by this exercise.

POSITIONING

- Take hold of a barbell with a shoulder-width grip, keeping your palms forward. Rest the barbell on your upper thighs.
- Keep your arms tightly pressed to your sides and stand in a natural position.
- Feel the weight of the barbell on your arms as you let it "hang" on your fingertips, your arms fully extended downward.

EXERCISE

- Slowly raise the barbell to your upper chest until it almost touches your chin. Flex your biceps and slowly return to starting position, letting the barbell stretch your arm. Allow the barbell to "hang" on your fingertips for a split second.
- Keep your wrists locked on the upward movement.
- Repeat the movement until you have completed the correct number of repetitions for your set.

ALERT

- Always flex on the upper movement and stretch on the downward movement.

"NEVERS"

- Never jerk the barbell up.
- Never let the barbell just drop because you are tired. Maintain control and concentrate at all times.
- Never hold your breath for a few repetitions. Relax and breathe naturally.
- Never let your wrists bend back on the upward movement. If you allow this, you will be doing the exercise with your shoulders and back instead of your biceps, and inefficiently at that. Your results will be greatly lessened. *Do the exercise in strict form.*

THE GYM WORKOUT **113**

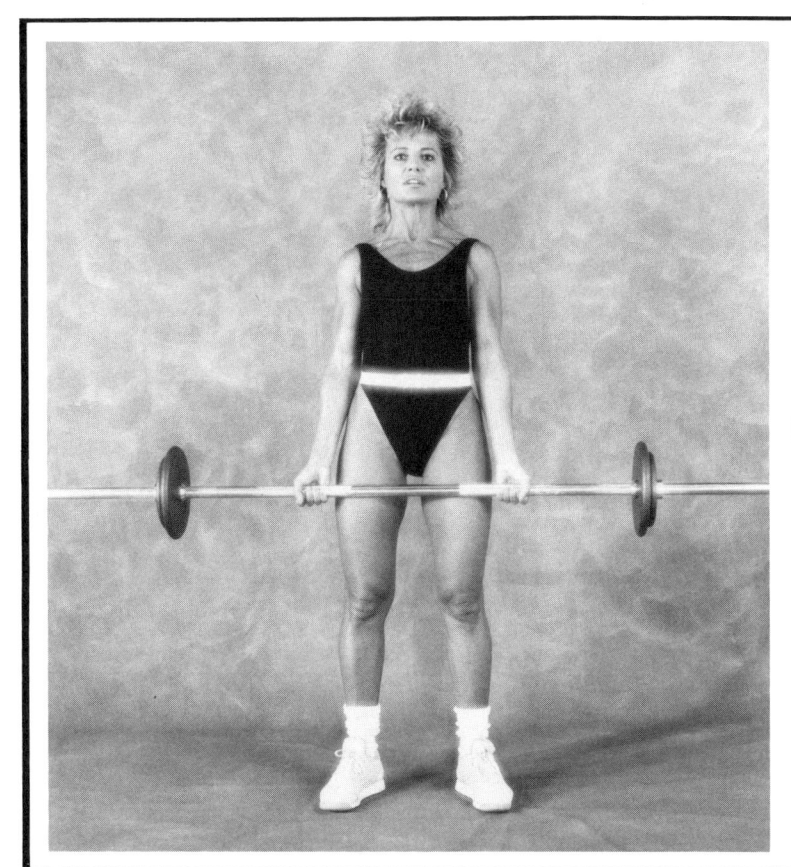

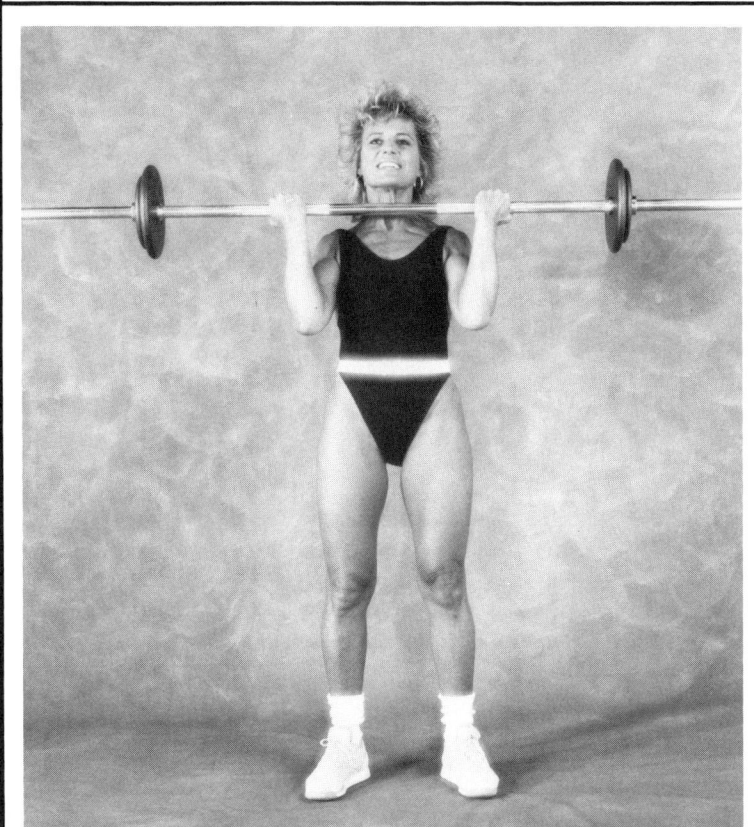

Start

Finish

One-Arm Preacher Curl— Biceps Exercise #2

The entire biceps is developed by this exercise, but the lower portion is especially stressed.

POSITIONING

- Hold a dumbbell in your right hand, so that the edge of the bench is directly under your armpit.
- Keep your left arm relaxed at your side and your right arm (with the dumbbell) fully extended over the bench surface.

EXERCISE

- Slowly raise your right arm, flexing as you do, until the dumbbell grazes your chin. Keep your wrist locked; do not ever let it bend back.
- Slowly lower the dumbbell to starting position, letting your biceps stretch out fully.
- Repeat the movement until you have performed the correct number of repetitions for your set.
- Repeat the set for your left arm.

ALERT

- Lean hard on the preacher's bench in order to isolate the biceps muscle and to ensure that no help is being given by other body parts.

"NEVERS"

- Never let the dumbbell drop into position.
- Never jerk the dumbbell up. Watch your chin.

THE GYM WORKOUT **115**

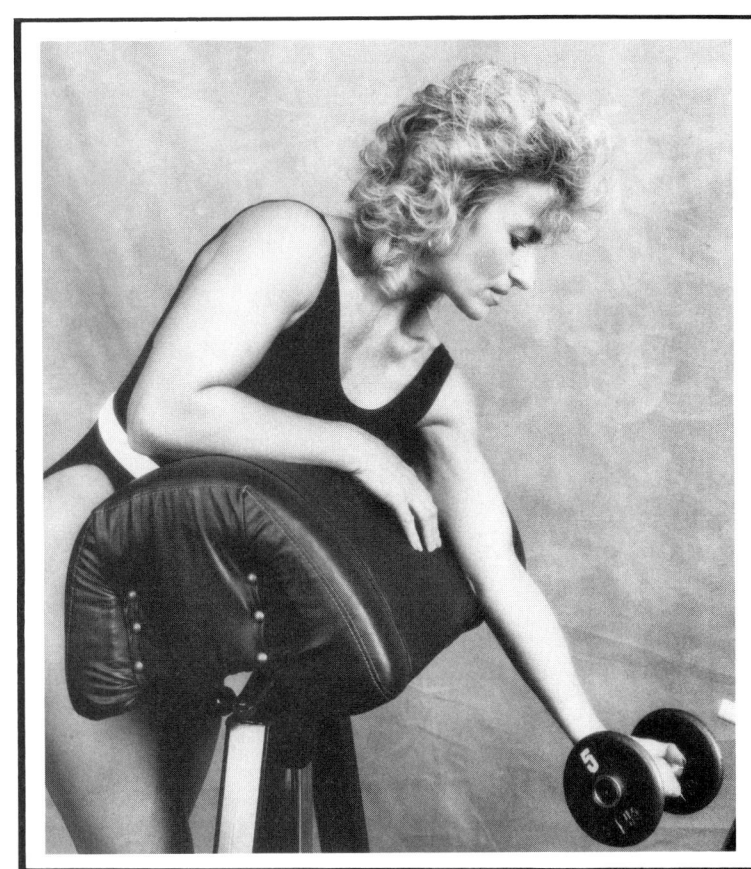

Start

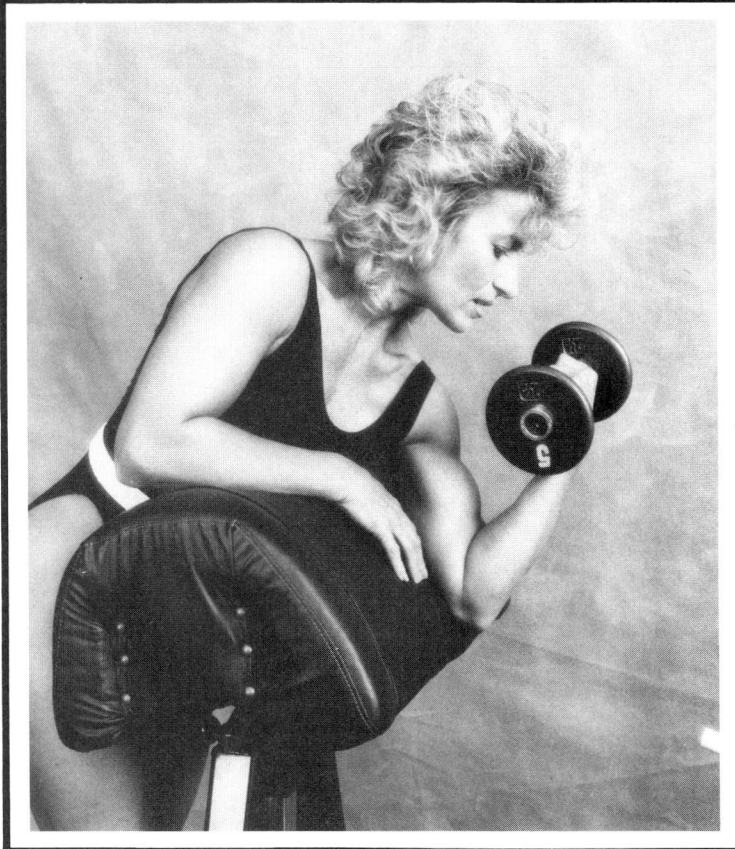

Finish

Concentration Curl—Biceps Exercise #3

The peak of your biceps muscle is developed by this exercise.

POSITIONING

- With a dumbbell in your right hand, sit on a flat exercise bench with your feet about two feet apart.
- Bend forward at the waist and place your right elbow on the inside of your right knee, holding the dumbbell with your palm facing outward.
- Allow the dumbbell to pull and stretch your right arm as the arm hangs straight down toward the floor.

EXERCISE

- Without bending your wrist, slowly raise the dumbbell by bending your elbow until the dumbbell nearly touches your chin. You should be leaning forward at all times during the exercise. Flex your biceps when your elbow is completely bent.
- Slowly lower the weight to starting position, maintaining control throughout the movement, and let the weight stretch out your arm and your biceps.
- Keeping your waist bent (do not sit up), repeat the movement until you have performed the correct number of repetitions for your set. Repeat the exercise for the other arm.

ALERT

- This exercise will require a light beginning weight and may take a little longer to get used to. Strict form in performance of the exercise is mandatory, so use a light weight and do the exercise exactly as instructed.

"NEVERS"

- Never jerk the weight up. You may hit yourself in the chin.
- Never let the weight just drop to the start position.
- Never sit up during the exercise.
- Never rest between alternating arms. One set constitutes separately working both arms. Quickly switch the dumbbell to the alternate arm and continue. There is also little reason to rest between sets (when one set of right and left arm has been completed), because the alternate arm has had a natural rest. Save time. Be intense. Move on.

THE GYM WORKOUT **117**

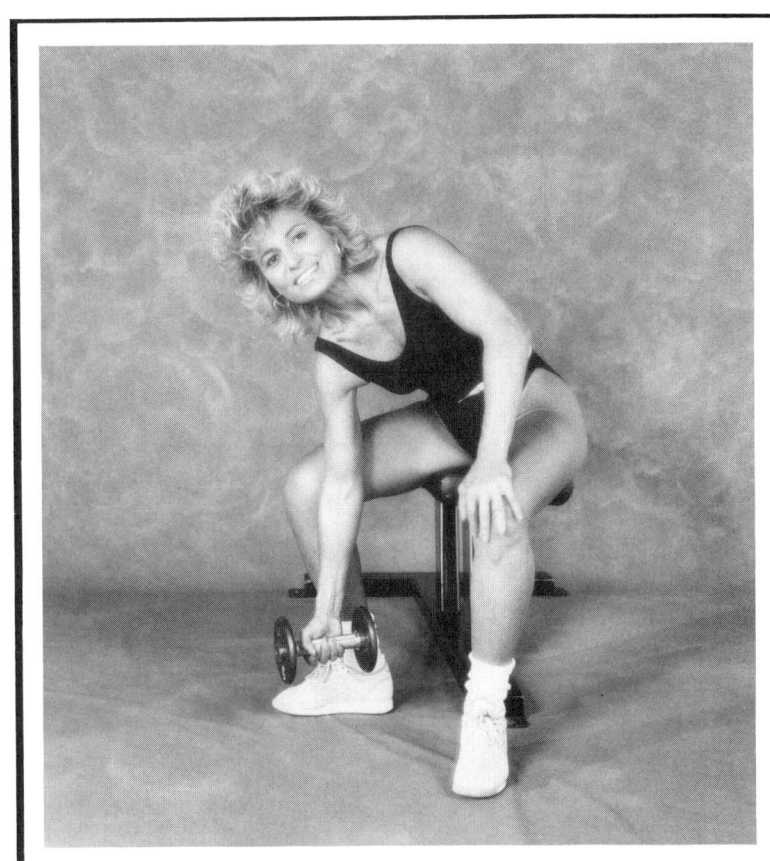

Start

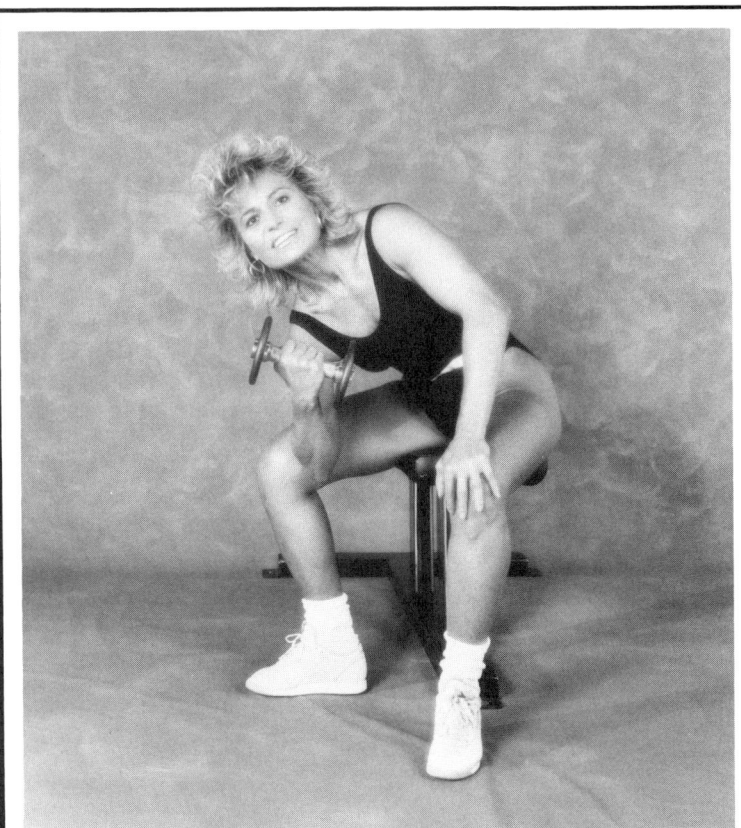

Finish

Incline Dumbbell Curl— Biceps Exercise #4

The entire biceps muscle is developed by this exercise.

POSITIONING

- Lie on an incline exercise bench with a dumbbell in each hand, palms held upward.
- Let your arms fall straight down near your sides.

EXERCISE

- Holding your arms close to your body throughout the exercise, slowly raise the dumbbells (both at the same time) in a semicircular motion until they reach your shoulders. Flex your biceps.
- Slowly return to starting position, letting your biceps fully stretch out, and repeat the movement until you have performed the correct number of repetitions for your set.

ALERT

- Alternate dumbbell curls can be performed instead, for variety. To do this, raise your right dumbbell, then as you lower it, raise your left dumbbell, and so on. The movement is a right, left, right, left movement, but don't wait until you have completed a full up-and-down movement with one arm to bring the other into play. Work both arms simultaneously.

"NEVERS"

- Never let your back rise from the bench in an arching movement made in an effort to give yourself leverage to jerk the weights into the up position. Keep your back flat against the bench at all times.
- Never let your arms just drop down in an effort to avoid the work of controlling the weights on the downward movement.

THE GYM WORKOUT **119**

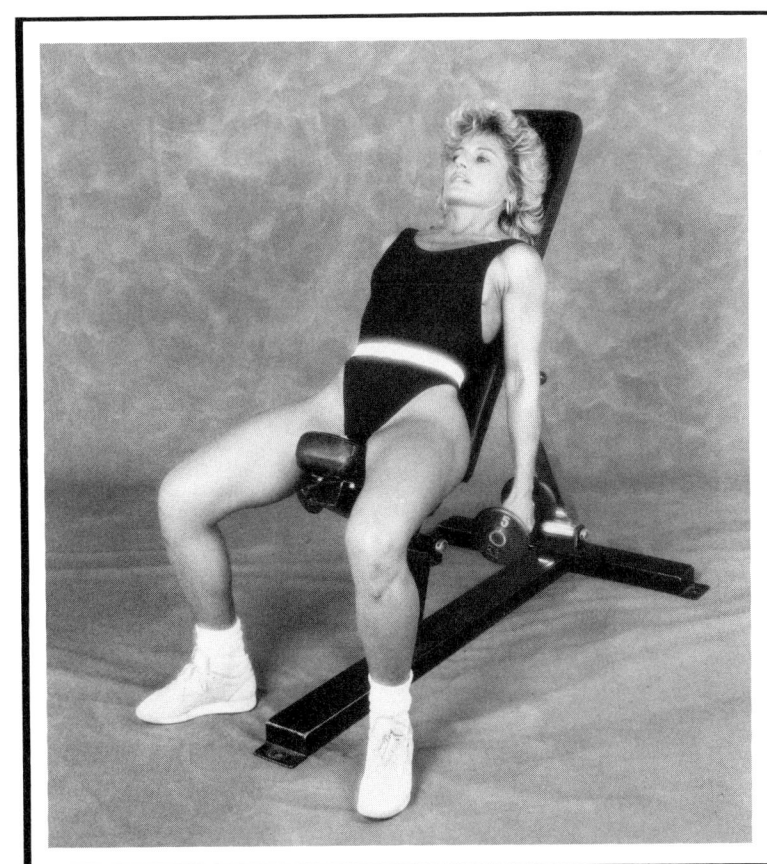

Start

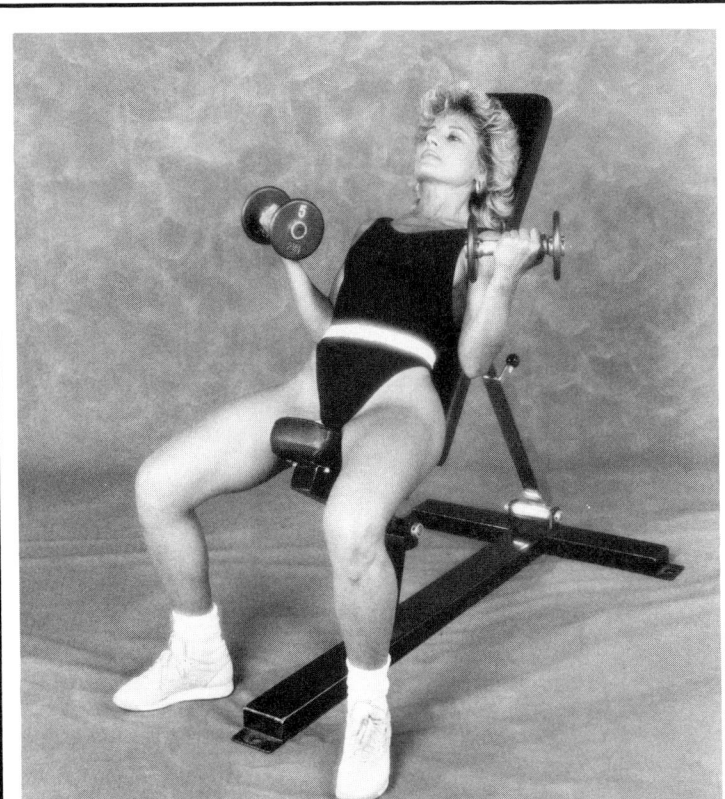

Finish

TRICEPS ROUTINE

One-Arm Dumbbell Triceps Extension— Triceps Exercise #1

The inner and middle points of the triceps muscle are stressed by this exercise.

POSITIONING

- Stand in front of a mirror with a dumbbell in your right hand.
- Raise your right arm straight up so that your biceps is touching your ear and your palm is facing the mirror.
- Place the other arm around the front of your waist for balance.

EXERCISE

- Maintaining control, slowly lower the dumbbell so that it moves down behind your head and touches the back of your neck.
- Return to the starting position and flex your triceps as you reach the highest point.
- Repeat the movement until you have performed the correct number of repetitions for your set.
- Repeat the set for your left arm.

ALERT

- Keep your biceps close to the side of your head as you perform the exercise.
- Be sure to move only the forearm from the elbow joint.

"NEVERS"

- Never let the dumbbell just drop down to your neck.
- Never place your fingers on your neck to assist in pushing off the dumbbell. You may smash your fingers. (I've done it.)

THE GYM WORKOUT **121**

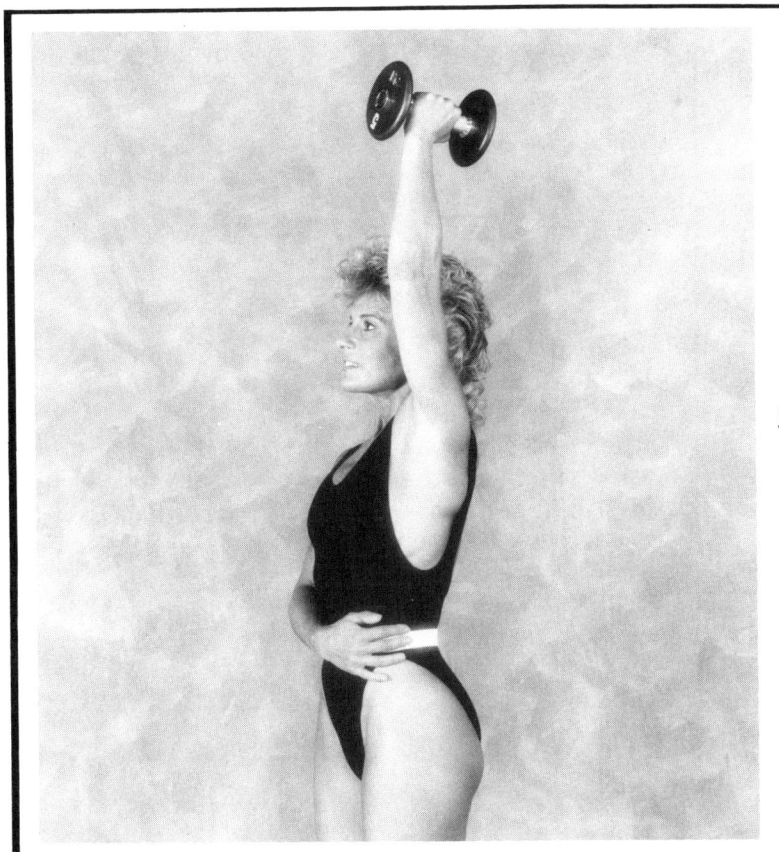

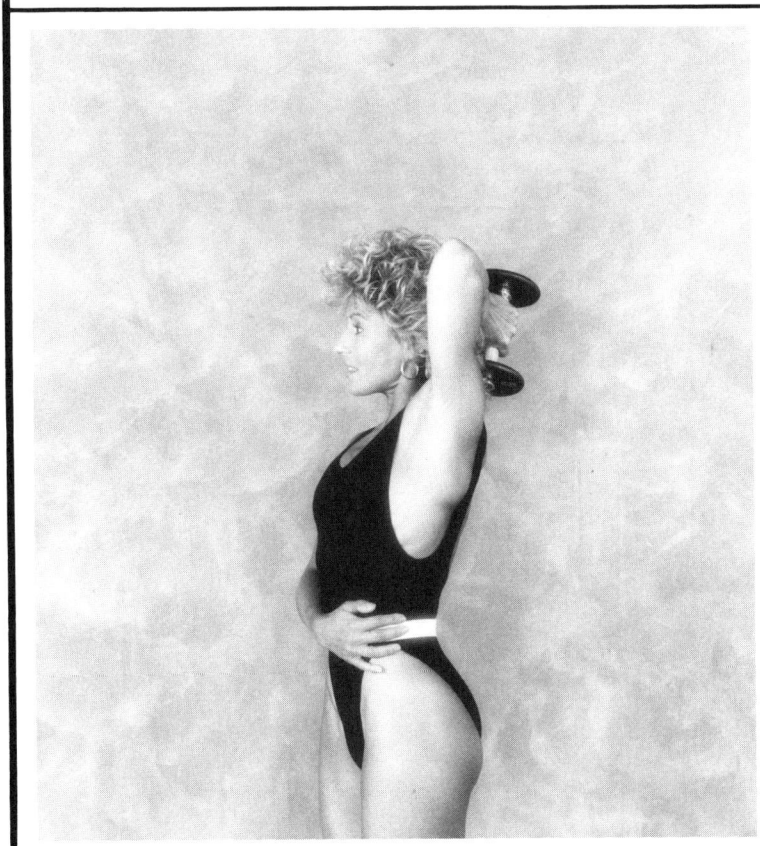

Start

Finish

Lying Triceps Extension—Triceps Exercise #2

The entire triceps area is developed by this exercise.

POSITIONING

- Take hold of a barbell, grasping it with hands held six inches apart from the middle of the barbell.
- Lie on a flat exercise bench and extend your arms upward. (Your palms should face away from you when the barbell is fully extended upward.) Hold the barbell directly above your chest. Keep your feet flat on the floor.

EXERCISE

- Keeping your upper arms still, slowly bend your elbows and, moving in an arclike motion, lower the barbell toward your forehead until the bar just grazes it.
- Slowly return to starting position and repeat the movement until you have performed the correct number of repetitions for your set.

ALERT

- You may vary the grip from time to time (from four to nine inches apart) in order to ensure development of every aspect of the triceps muscle.

"NEVERS"

- Never let your elbows wander outward from your body.
- Never let the barbell just drop toward your forehead in an effort to remove stress from the working triceps. Control the barbell at all times.
- Never cut your movements short. Raise the barbell until your arms are fully extended, and lower it until it nearly touches your forehead.
- Never hold your breath for a few repetitions. Breathe naturally.

THE GYM WORKOUT **123**

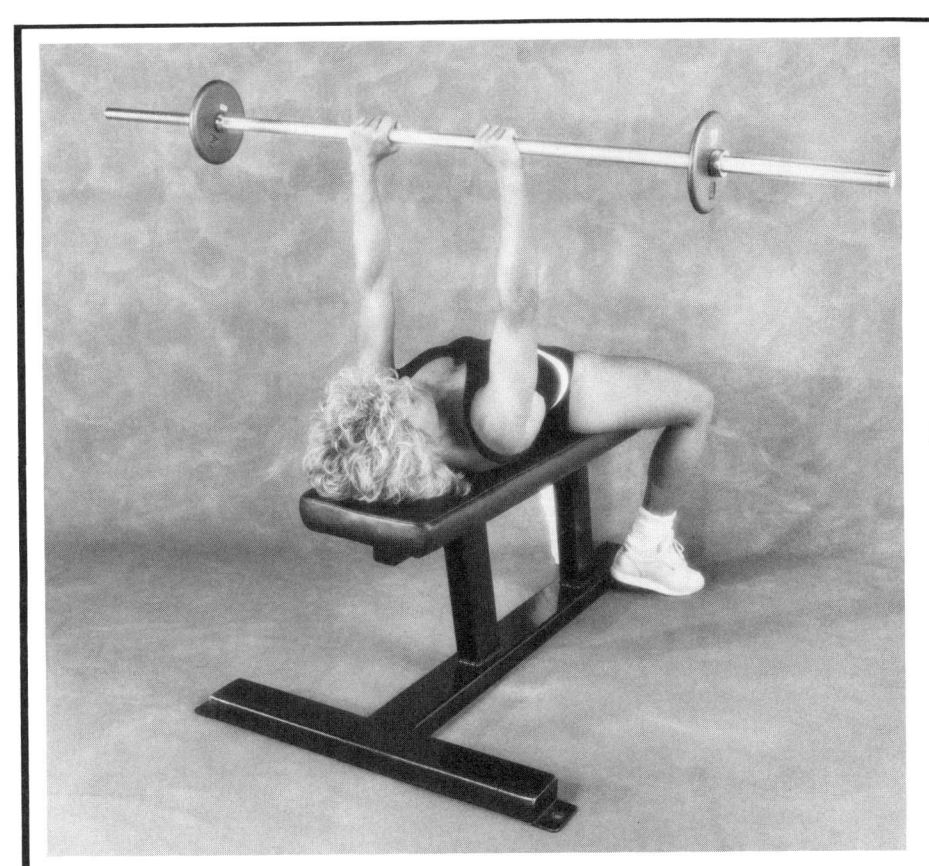

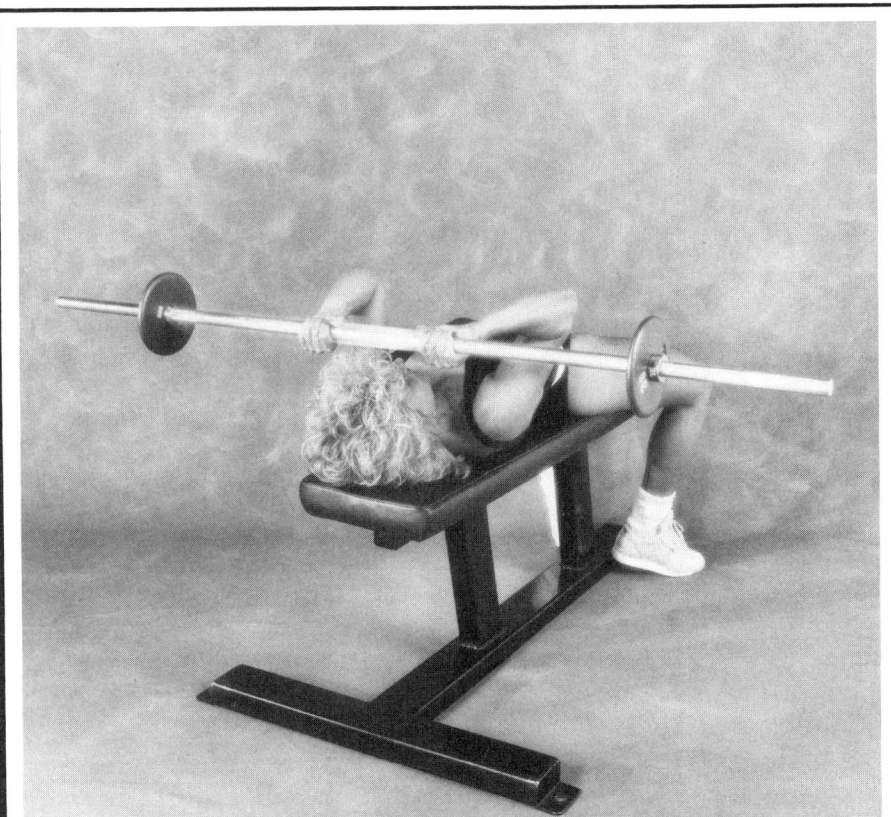

Start

Finish

Pulley Pushdown—Triceps Exercise #3

The entire triceps area is worked by this exercise. It may be performed on any appropriate gym machine. It is described here for the free-standing pulley.

POSITIONING

- Place the curved pulley pushdown bar on the pulley and hold the bar with a hand on either side of it.
- Bend at the elbows and fully extend your forearms upward.
- Keep your upper arms pinned to your body throughout the exercise.

EXERCISE

- Slowly lower the bar until your arms are fully extended downward. Flex your triceps.
- Maintaining full control, slowly return to starting position.
- Repeat the movement until you have performed the correct number of repetitions for your set.

ALERT

- You may use a straight bar if a curved bar is not available.

"NEVERS"

- Never jerk the bar down. If the weight is too heavy, reduce it.
- Never let the weight just pull your arms up to starting position. Control the weight at all times.
- Never let your elbows wander away from your upper body.

THE GYM WORKOUT **125**

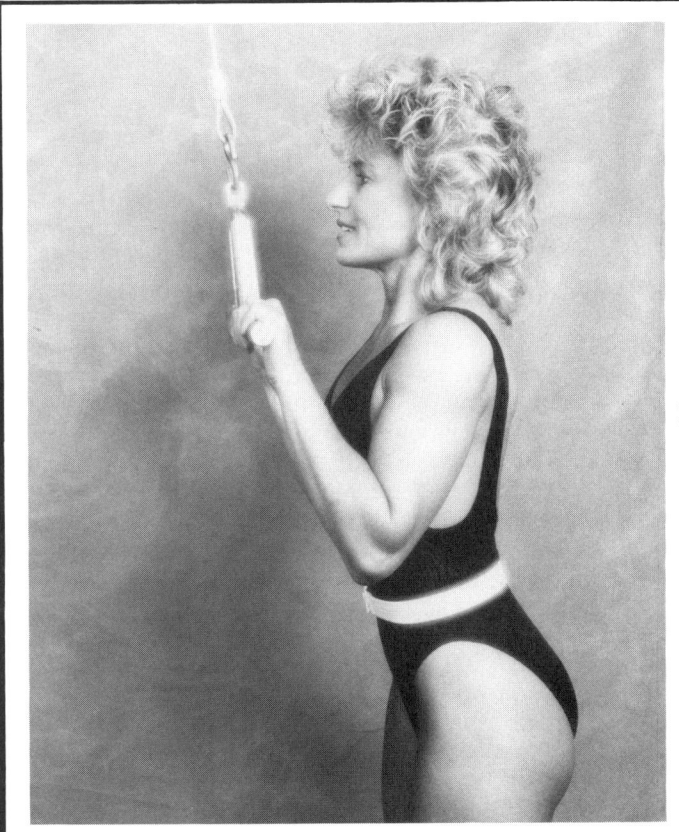

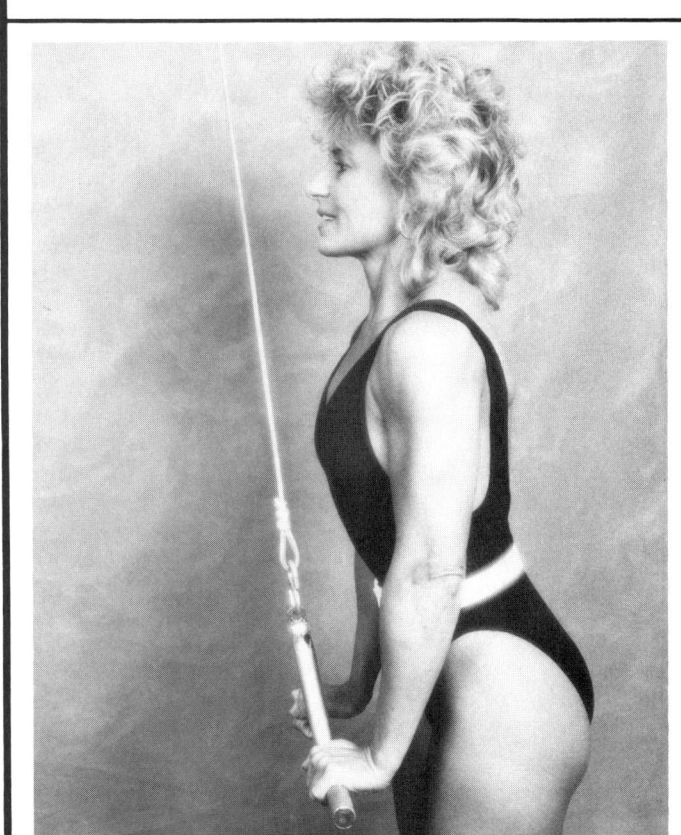

Start

Finish

Dips between Benches—Triceps Exercise #4

The entire triceps muscle is developed by this exercise.

POSITIONING

- Line up two flat exercise benches so that they are parallel to each other and wide enough apart so that when you lean on one with the palms of your hands the heels of your feet just fit on the edge of the other one without falling off. If another exercise bench is not available, you may pile up blocks of wood or use any other device to support your heels. Keep the heel rest either at the same height as the arm rest or a little higher.
- Curl your fingers around the edge of the bench, holding your hands about four to six inches apart.

EXERCISE

- Slowly lower your body as far down as possible by bending your upper arms. Keep your triceps flexed. Think about those muscles.
- Return to starting position and immediately repeat the movement until you have performed the correct number of repetitions for your set.
- You should return to starting position (the up position) at about twice the speed at which you lowered yourself (to the down position).

ALERT

- This exercise should seem almost impossible to perform at first. Don't despair. Do it even if you can manage only one or two reps. As your triceps strengthen, you will find it easier to do the exercise.
- Notice that no weight is used for this exercise. You may still do less reps for succeeding sets, but if you wish, you can do fifteen repetitions for each set. (It may take about six months to achieve that ability.)
- If you find it utterly impossible to manage even one repetition, take a wider grip (about shoulder width) and perform the exercise that way. If it is still impossible for you to get even one repetition, you may place your heels on the ground instead of on an exercise bench. After a month you will be able to get a few reps placing your feet on the bench. Everything in time.
- I don't advise it, but if you really hate this exercise, you may substitute dumbbell kickbacks in its place (see page 174).

"NEVERS"

- Never cut the movement short by lowering and raising yourself a mere two inches.
- Never rest when you return to starting position. *Keep going.*
- Never give up. Eventually you will get this down to a science.

THE GYM WORKOUT **127**

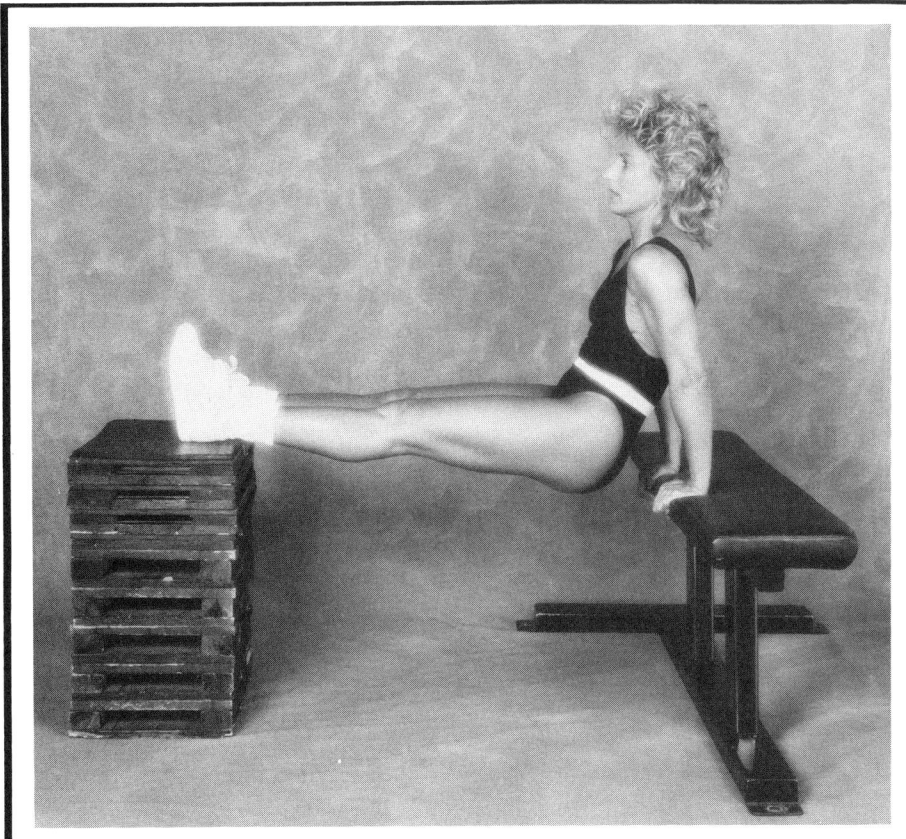

Start

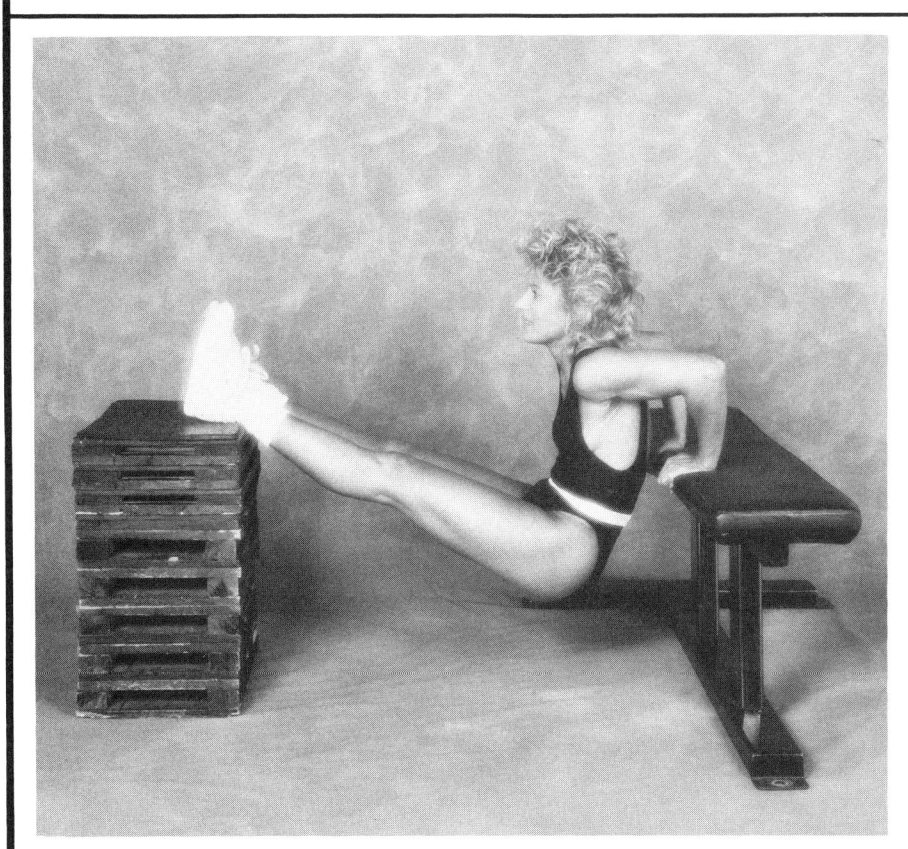

Finish

LEG ROUTINE

Lunge—Leg Exercise #1

The entire front thigh (quadriceps) muscle is developed by this exercise, and the buttocks (gluteus maximus) is tightened and strengthened as well.

POSITIONING

- With a barbell placed across your shoulders and resting on your trapezius muscles, stand with feet shoulder width apart and point your toes in a natural position.

EXERCISE

- Keeping your left leg straight, step forward with your right foot and, bending your right knee as you do so, lower your body as far as possible.
- Keep your torso from leaning forward by looking straight ahead into a mirror.
- Continue the movement until your left knee grazes the floor and then slowly, without lurching, return to starting position.
- Repeat the movement for the left leg and continue this right-left movement until you have completed the correct number of repetitions for your set.

ALERT

- Be sure to stretch the quadriceps muscles as you take the down position (the forward lunge). You should feel the muscle pulling.
- You may feel awkward at first. If you always return to your exact starting position, you will be able to set up a balance and rhythm.

"NEVERS"

- Never use a towel or a rubber pad for your shoulders. This is an unnecessary "crutch" and symbolizes weakness. Your trapezius muscles are pads. Use them.
- Never bounce off your leg. Rather, maintain control as you rise up, using your quadriceps muscles.

THE GYM WORKOUT 129

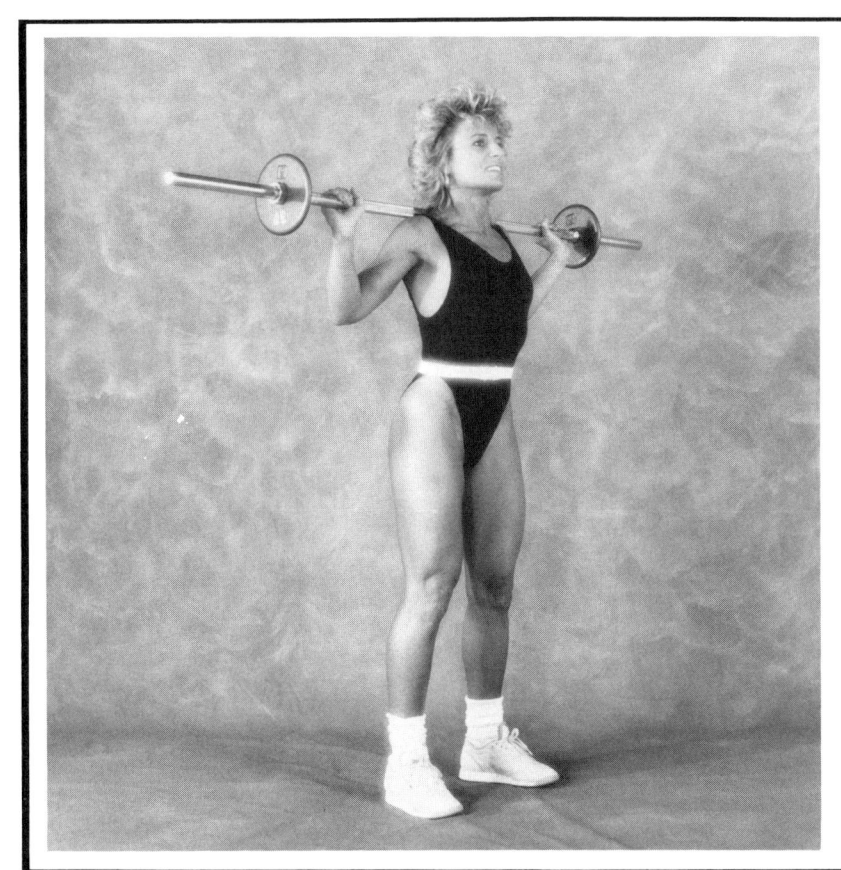

Start

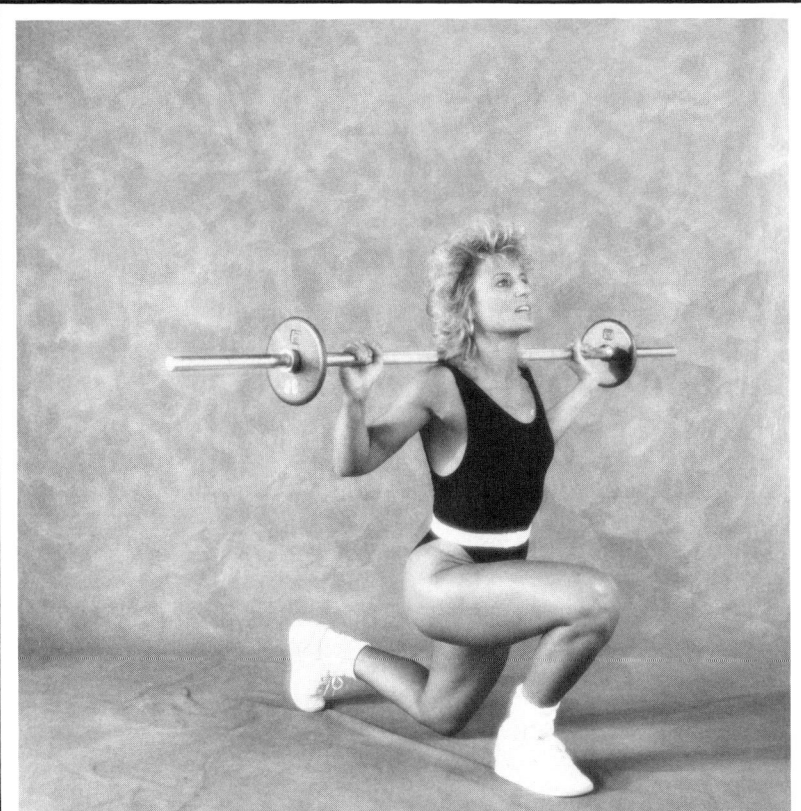

Finish

Squat—Leg Exercise #2

The front thigh muscles (quadriceps) are developed by this exercise, and the buttocks (gluteus maximus) is tightened as well.

POSITIONING

- Place a light barbell across your shoulders, balancing it on your trapezius muscles.
- Stand with your feet shoulder width apart and your toes pointing out at about a 45° angle to each side.
- Flex your abdominal muscles and stand straight. Look into the mirror directly ahead, focusing on a set point so that you keep your head and back erect throughout the exercise. Be careful not to let your buttocks jut out. Keep your buttocks in direct line with the heels of your feet.

EXERCISE

- Slowly lower yourself into a squatting position by bending at the knees. As you are bending, be sure to keep your knees in direct line with your feet. (Your knees should move out in line with your feet.)
- Descend as low as your knees will allow, then slowly rise to starting position. Throw your mind into your quadriceps muscle. Be sure that it is your quadriceps (thigh muscle) that is doing the work.
- Repeat the movement, flexing on the upward position and stretching on the downward position, until you have performed the correct number of repetitions for your set.

ALERT

- You may place a two-by-four piece of wood under your heels if this makes it easier to maintain balance.
- You may vary the position of your toes for each of your three sets: Position One, as above; Position Two, toes angled outward as far as possible; Position Three, feet close together, toes straight ahead. This changing of the toe position ensures well-rounded development of the quadriceps.

"NEVERS"

- Never bounce off the lowest point of the movement in an attempt to gain momentum to rise to the starting position. Instead use the strength of the quadriceps muscle to elevate you slowly.
- Never hold your breath for a few repetitions. Remember to breathe naturally. You may want to inhale on the down movement and exhale on the up movement. However, it is better just to breathe naturally.

THE GYM WORKOUT **131**

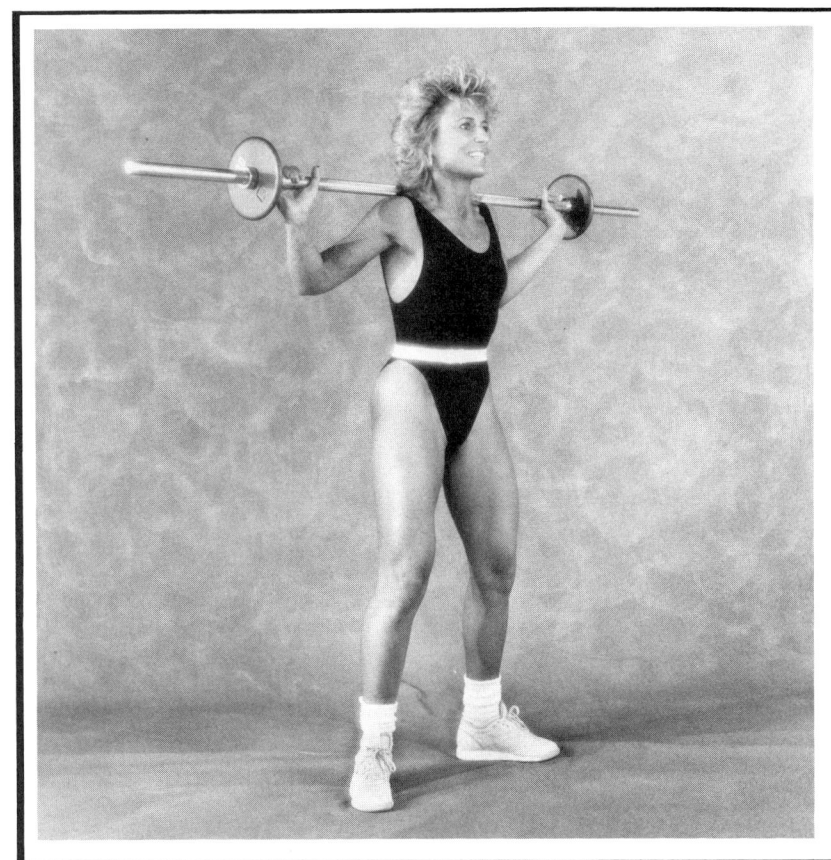

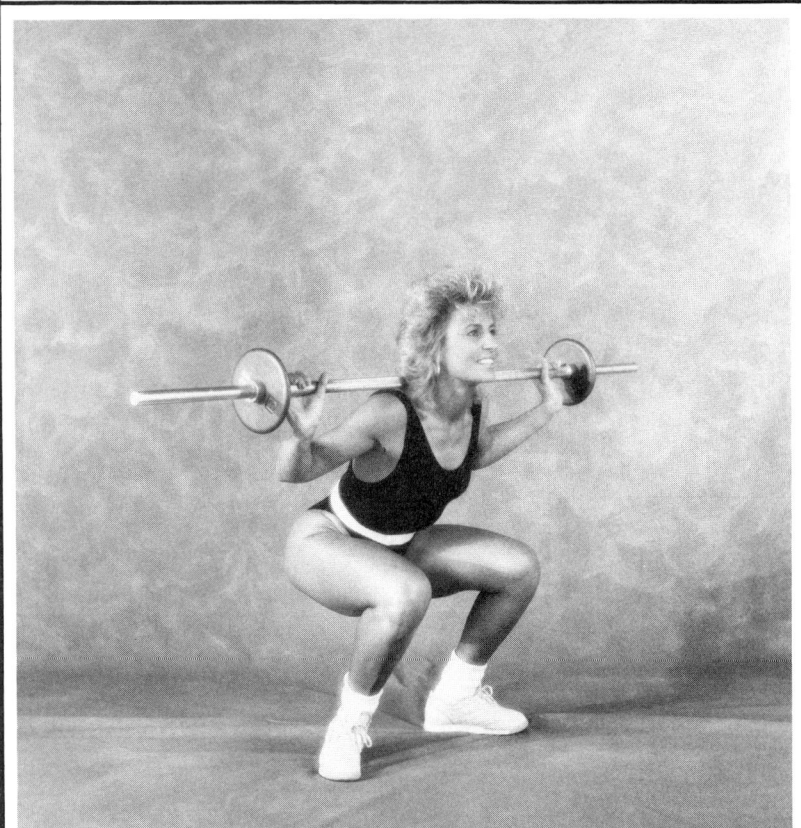

Start

Finish

Leg Extension—Leg Exercise #3

The front thigh (quadriceps) muscle is developed by this exercise. It can be done on any appropriate gym machine.

POSITIONING

- Sit in the machine seat and place your insteps under the machine roller pad.
- Hold on to the handles or the side of the seat on either side of you.

EXERCISE

- Slowly extend your legs until they are straight out in front of you, and hold that position for a split second. Flex.
- Maintaining full control, return to starting position. Repeat the movement until you have performed the correct number of repetitions for your set.

ALERT

- As you perform the movement, watch your quadriceps expand and contract. Mentally tell your muscle to take the shape you picture as ideal.

"NEVERS"

- Never bounce the weight up.
- Never let the roller pad just drop down because you are tired. Instead maintain full control through the repeated movements until you complete your set.

THE GYM WORKOUT **133**

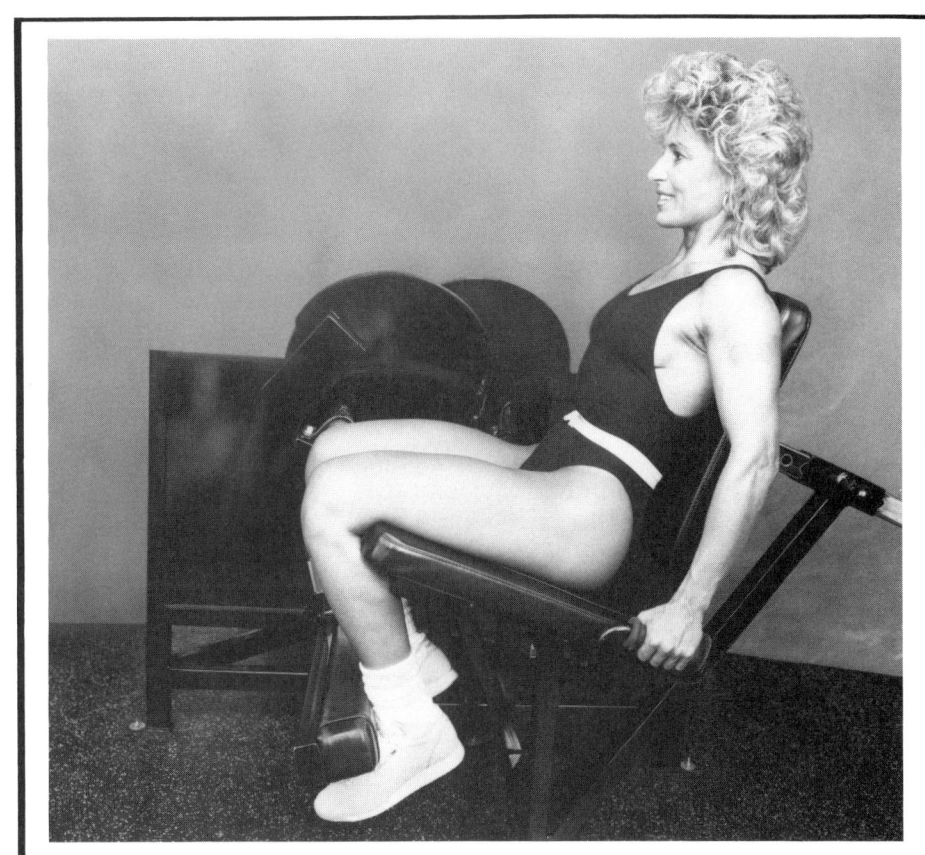

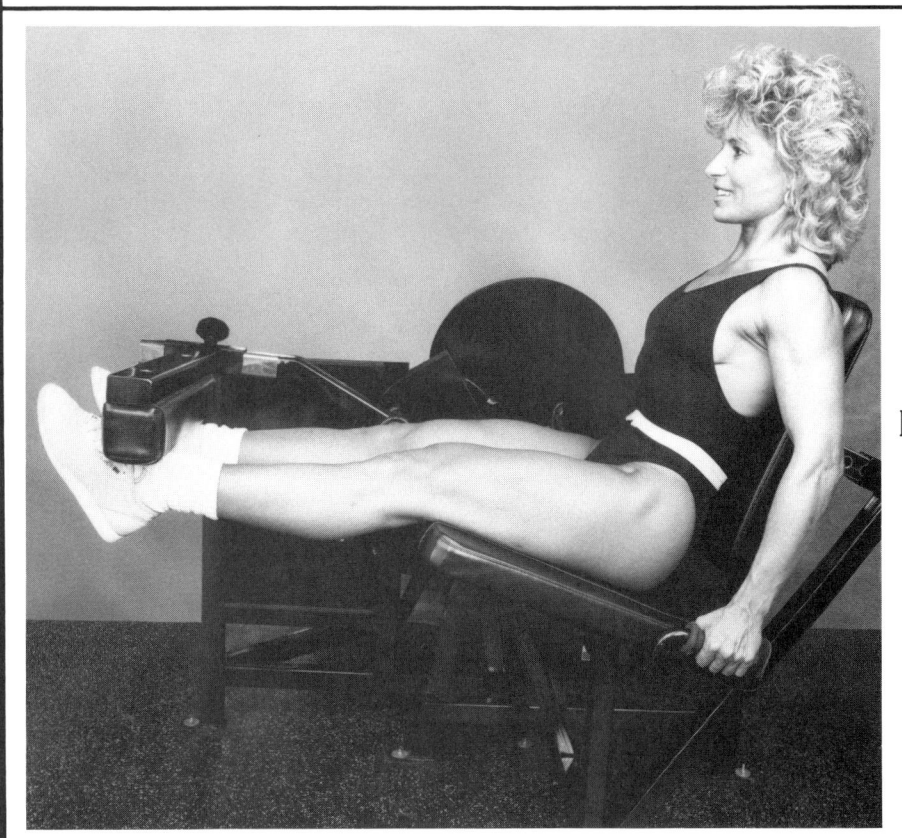

Start

Finish

Leg Curl—Leg Exercise #4

The back thigh (biceps femoris, or hamstring) muscles are developed by this exercise. It can be performed on any appropriate gym machine.

POSITIONING

- Lie on the padded surface (table) facedown.
- Place your heels under the roller pads and hold on to the handles or the table edge on either side of you.

EXERCISE

- Slowly bend your legs at the knee, raising your feet upward until your legs are perpendicular to the floor.
- Hold the position for a split second and, maintaining control, return to starting position. Flex your back thighs.
- Repeat the movement until you have performed the correct number of repetitions for your set.

ALERT

- Concentrate on your back thighs as you do the exercise and picture the muscle taking shape. Mentally see the excess fat being worn away from your hamstring area.

"NEVERS"

- Never let your back rise from the table in an arch.
- Never let your abdomen leave the table surface.
- Never swing the weight up.
- Never drop the weight down. Control it at all times.

THE GYM WORKOUT **135**

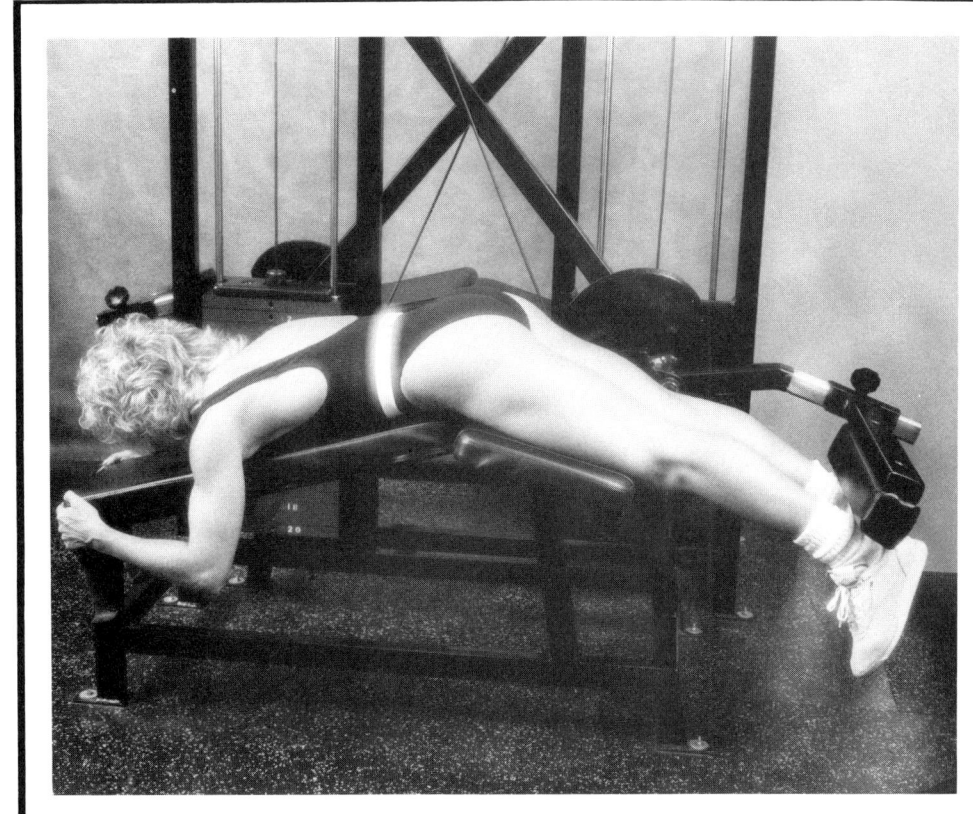

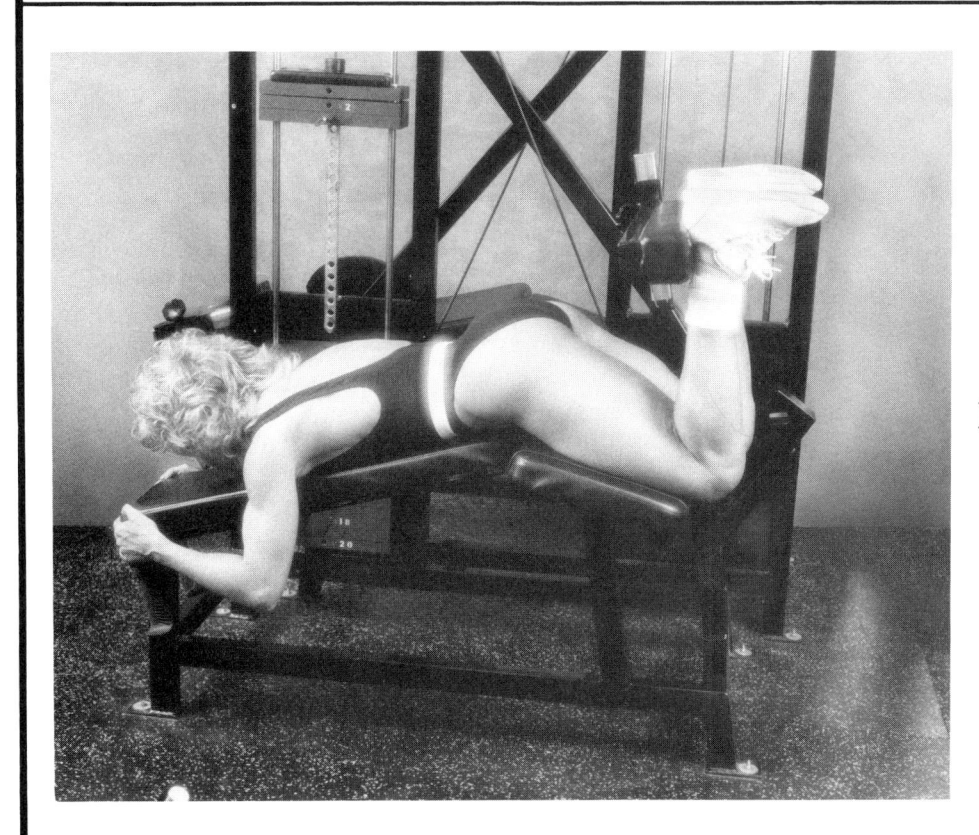

Start

Finish

One-Leg Toe Raise— Leg Exercise #5

The calf muscles (gastrocnemius) are developed by this exercise.

POSITIONING

- Stand on a block of wood that is about eight inches high.
- Grasp a dumbbell (about twenty pounds) in your right hand.
- Place the ball of your right foot on the edge of the block, letting your heel and arch extend off the wood.
- Be sure that your left foot is not touching the block of wood.
- Stand on your right toe, raising yourself as high as possible.
- Use your arms to hold on to a convenient object for balance.

EXERCISE

- Slowly lower your right heel toward the floor as you stretch your calf muscle. Be sure to lower your heel to the greatest possible extent.
- Ascend slowly to starting position and repeat the movement until you have performed the correct number of repetitions for your set.

ALERT

- Some gyms have a calf machine, which produces the same results as this exercise. On the machine, both calves are worked at the same time. You may use that machine in lieu of this exercise if you wish.

"NEVERS"

- Never shorten the length of the drop when lowering your heel. Stretch the calf muscle on the downward move and flex it on the upward move. Picture your calf muscle taking shapely form.
- Never shorten the height of the ascent. Be sure to rise up to the tip of your toe.

THE GYM WORKOUT **137**

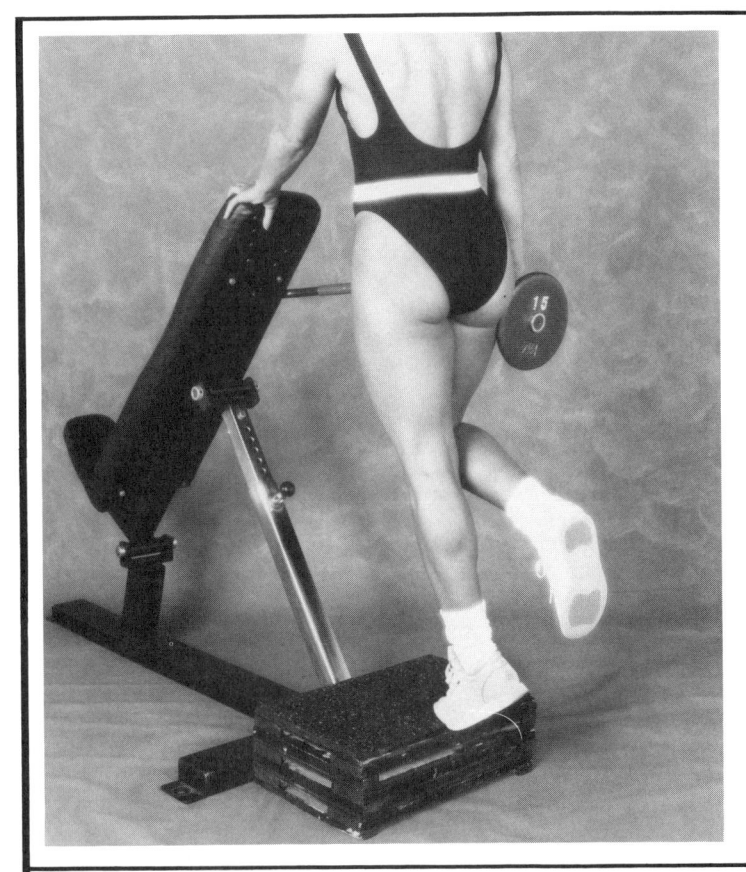

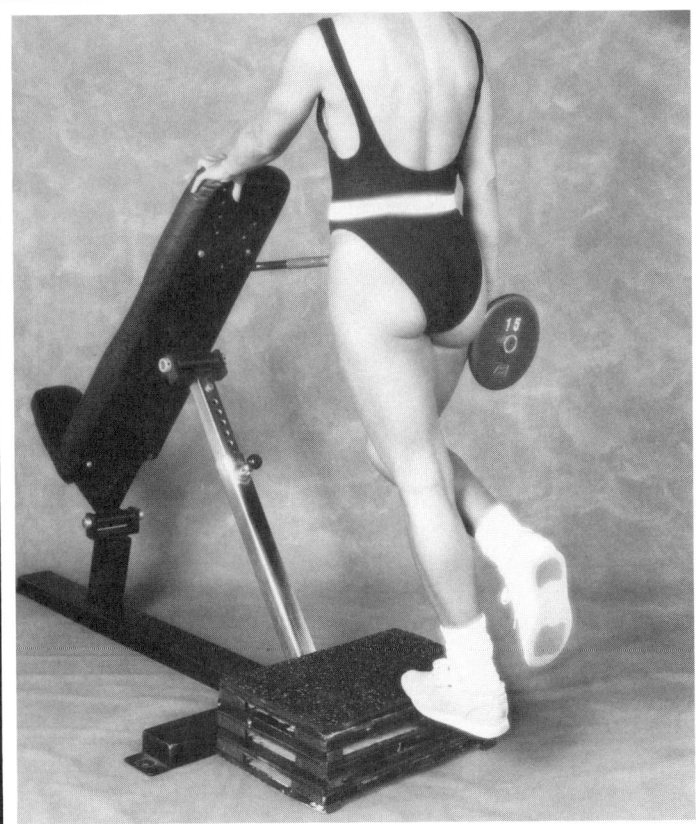

Start

Finish

ABDOMINAL ROUTINE

The abdominal area requires more work than other body parts, so you will do more repetitions. You will do twenty-five repetitions for each exercise. You may start with ten repetitions and add one repetition each week until you are up to twenty-five repetitions. If you are more ambitious, you may even go as high as fifty repetitions per set. Even champion bodybuilders work their abdominal areas harder than other body parts.

Since no real gym equipment is needed to perform the abdominal routine, some women work their abdominals at home in the morning, before going to the gym. This saves them about fifteen minutes of gym time. (You can do the same for your buttocks routine, netting you a total time saving of a half hour in the gym. This can be very convenient if you are in a hurry that day.)

The abdominals are worked every workout day.

DAYS ONE, TWO, THREE, AND FOUR

Straight and Incline Sit-ups— Abdominal Exercise #1

This exercise develops the upper half of the abdominal muscles (above the waist) and slightly stresses the lower abdominals (below the waist).

POSITIONING
- Lie flat on your back on a padded sit-up board. (The board may be placed on the floor or placed on an incline.)
- Place your feet under the leather strap or roller pad.
- Bend your knees slightly and cross your arms in front of you, or place them behind your head.

EXERCISE
- Slowly raise yourself from a prone position, curling yourself upward until you are perpendicular to the board.
- Without hesitation, slowly return to starting position and repeat the movement until you have performed the correct number of repetitions for your set.

ALERT
- Flex (squeeze) your abdominals (lower and upper) throughout the movement.
- You may wedge your feet under a heavy piece of furniture and lie on the floor if you are doing your sit-ups at home.

"NEVERS"
- Never bounce off the board. Instead, slowly raise and lower yourself.

NOTE
- Do your abdominal work on a flat board for the first few weeks. Once you have achieved three sets of twenty-five repetitions, you may raise the board to an incline. You can increase the incline as the exercise becomes easier.

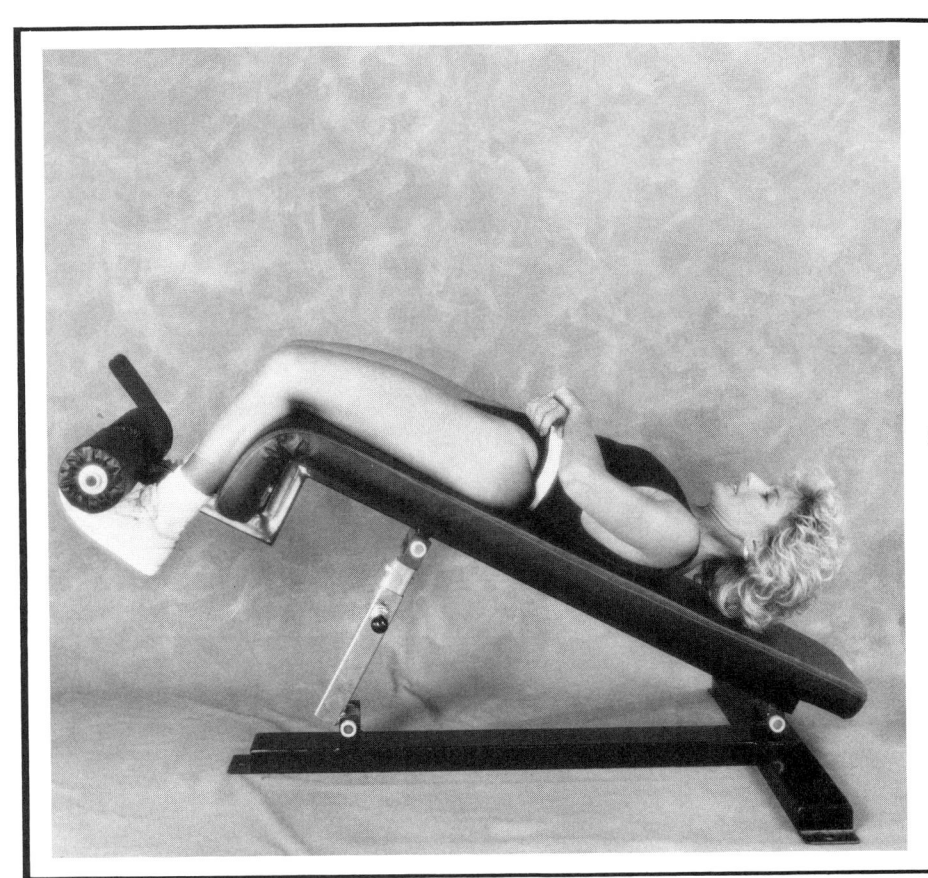

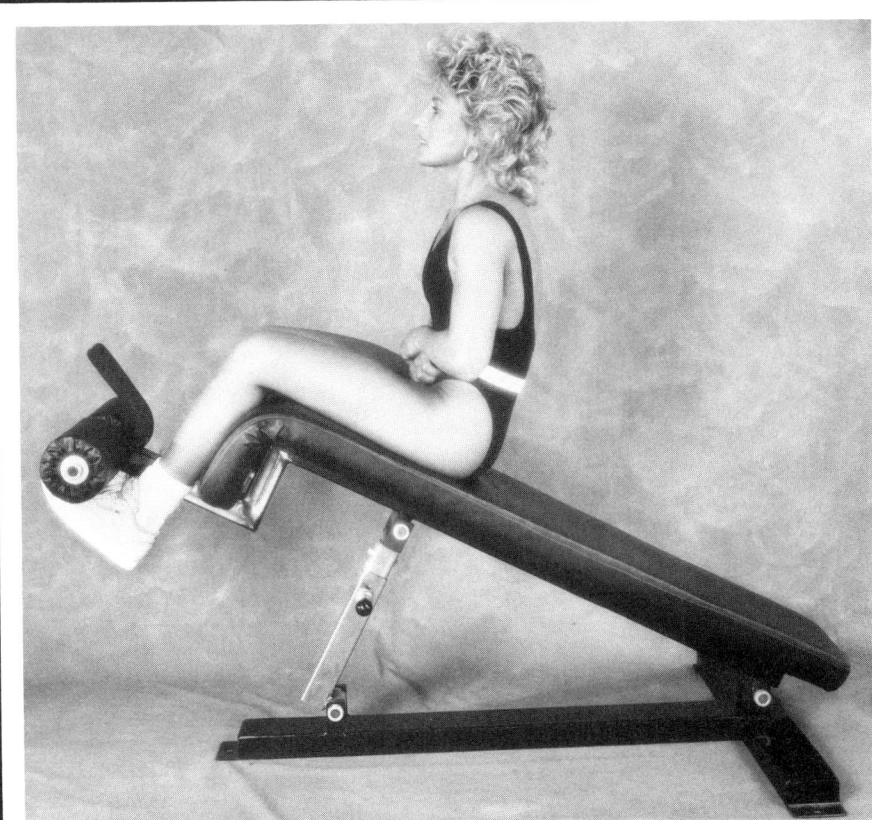

Start

Finish

Crunch—Abdominal Exercise #2

The upper abdominals are developed by this exercise.

POSITIONING

- Lie on the floor on your back and place your legs, crossed, over a flat exercise bench.
- Be sure that your legs are at an approximate 90° angle.
- Fold your hands behind your neck.

EXERCISE

- Slowly curl your body up, using only your shoulders and upper abdominals to do the work.
- Rise only high enough to lift your entire shoulder area off the floor. Do not go higher.
- Slowly lower yourself to starting position and, without resting for even a split second, repeat the movement until you have performed the correct number of repetitions for your set.

ALERT

- Flex your abdominal muscles throughout the movement.
- Mentally picture your upper abdominals being formed.

"NEVERS"

- Never lurch off the floor.
- Never raise yourself higher than necessary to lift your shoulders off the floor level.
- Never rest when you return to start position.
- Never hold your breath for a few repetitions. Breathe naturally.

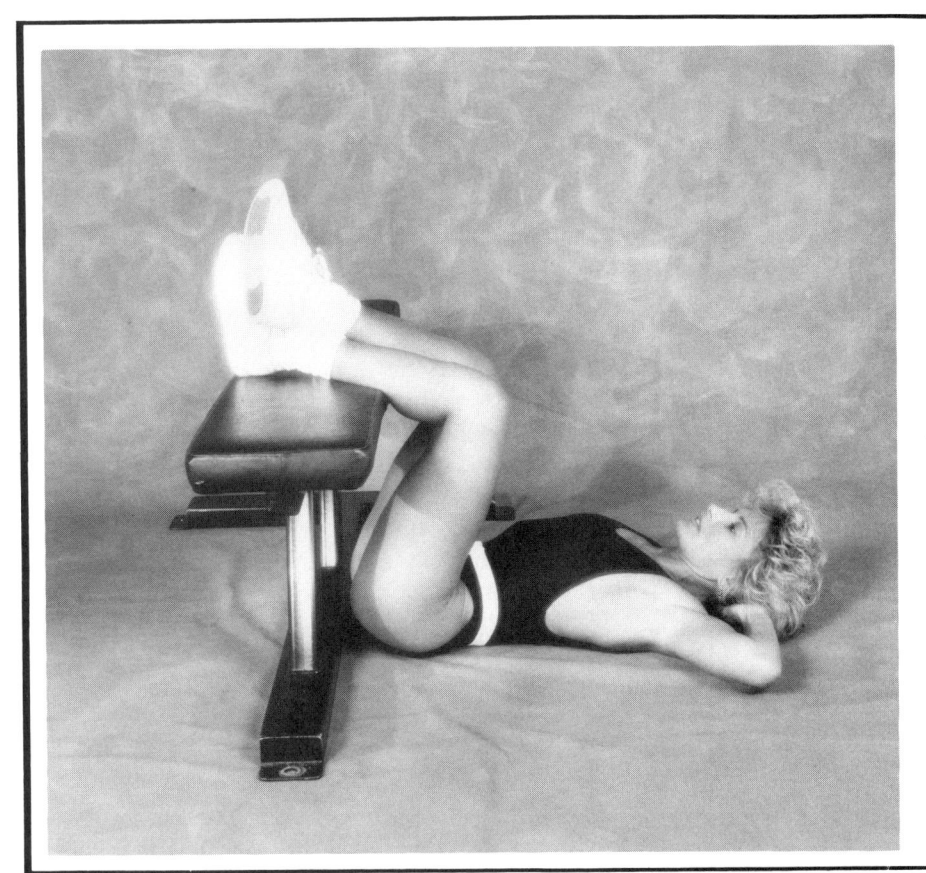

THE GYM WORKOUT 141

Start

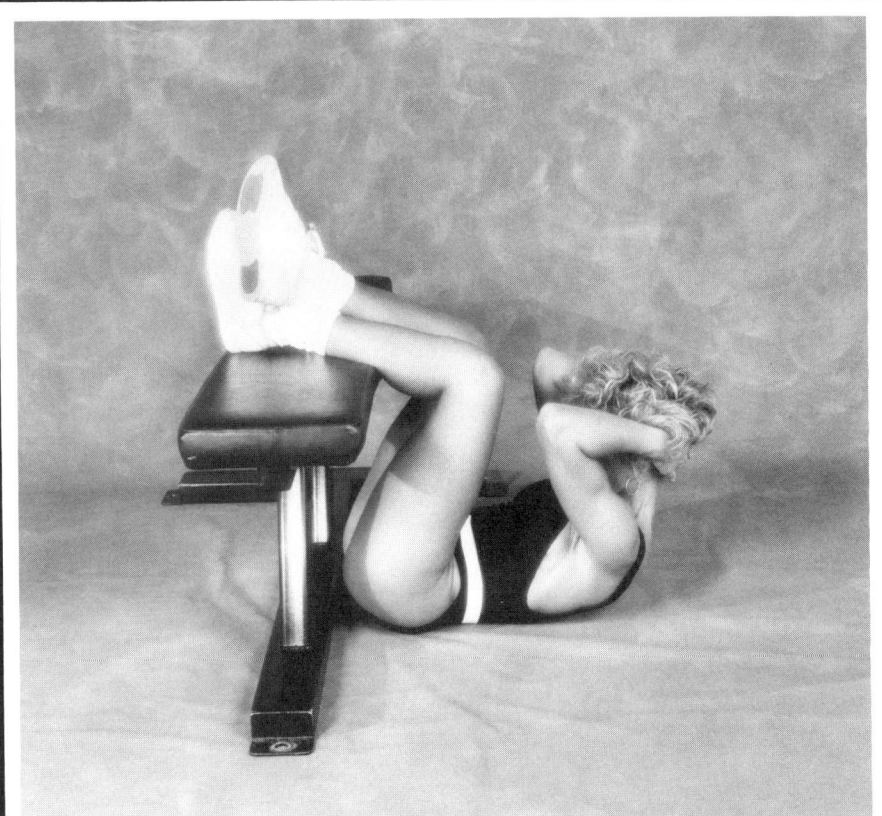

Finish

Bench Leg Raise with and without a Weight—Abdominal Exercise #3

This exercise develops the lower abdominal muscles. It is described here using a weight. Begin doing the exercise for the first month without the weight, following the directions exactly, omitting only the weight. After a month, add a light weight (about five pounds).

POSITIONING

- Place a light weight between your ankles as you lie on a flat exercise bench or a floorboard.
- Keep your back flat to the surface and your hips touching the end of the board or bench.
- Hold on to the board or bench on either side near your hips and bend your knees slightly. (You may place your hands under your buttocks on either side if you wish instead of holding on to the board or bench.)

EXERCISE

- With knees very slightly bent, slowly raise your legs until they are perpendicular to the floor, then slowly lower them to starting position.
- Without resting for even a split second, repeat the movement until you have performed the correct number of repetitions for your set. Keep your abdominal muscles flexed at all times.
- After your last set, hold your legs six inches off the floor for thirty seconds. (Begin with five seconds and work up to thirty seconds.)

ALERT

- Keep a mental grip on the weight. It is dangerous to let your mind wander. The weight can fall on you and hurt your face.

"NEVERS"

- Never raise the weight in a fast, abrupt movement. Instead, slowly raise your legs while maintaining complete control.
- Never let your legs just drop down to starting position.

THE GYM WORKOUT 143

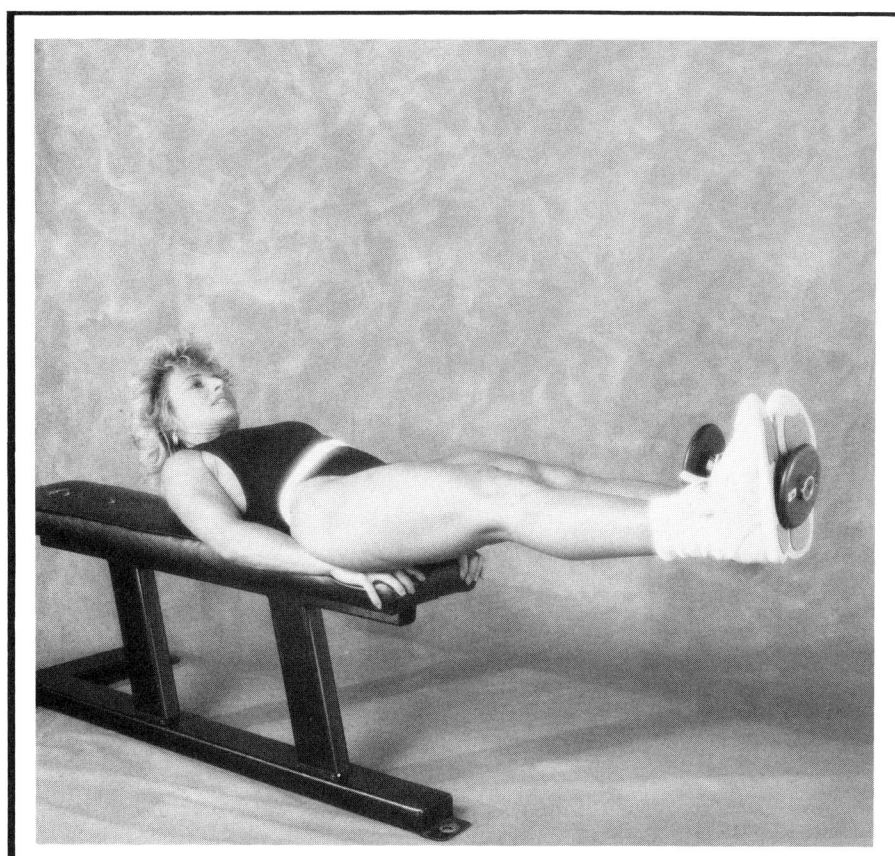

Start

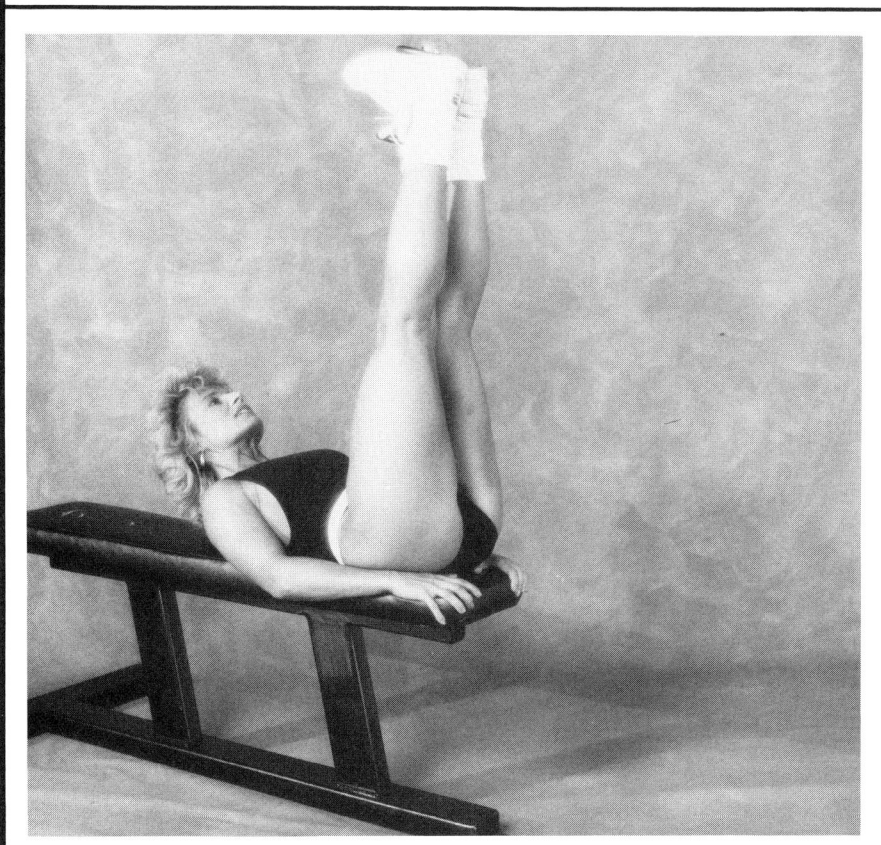

Finish

Leg-in with and without a Weight— Abdominal Exercise #4

This exercise develops the lower abdominal area. It is described here with a weight. Begin the exercise for the first month without a weight, following the directions exactly, omitting only the weight. After a month, add a light weight (about five pounds).

POSITIONING

- Lie on a flat exercise bench, your buttocks on the bench but your legs completely off the bench.
- Place a light weight between your feet.
- Grasp the bench on either side of you.
- Keeping your back flat on the bench—you may raise your head to see your legs working—extend your legs straight out.

EXERCISE

- Slowly bring your knees as close to your chest as possible.
- Immediately return to starting position, keeping your abdominals flexed at all times.
- Without resting for even a split second, repeat the movement until you have performed the correct number of repetitions for your set.

ALERT

- Be aware of the weight at all times. Hold it securely.

"NEVERS"

- Never rush the exercise. Tuck and extend your legs slowly.
- Never let your mind wander—you could catapult the weight onto your face.

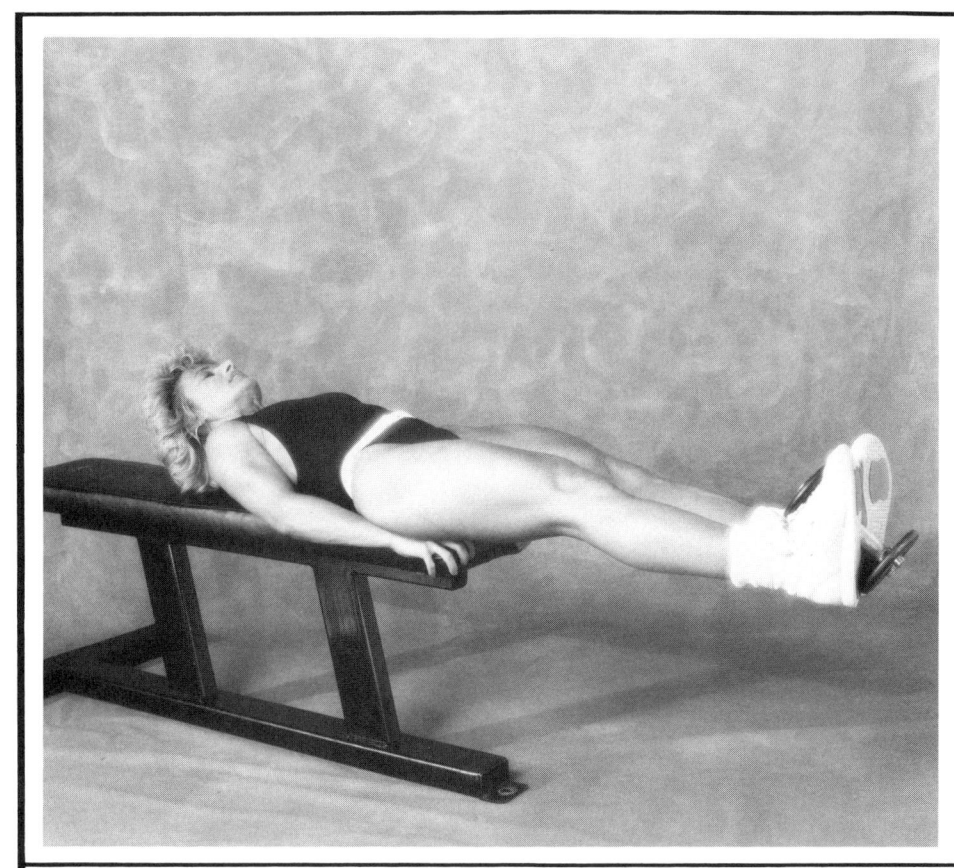

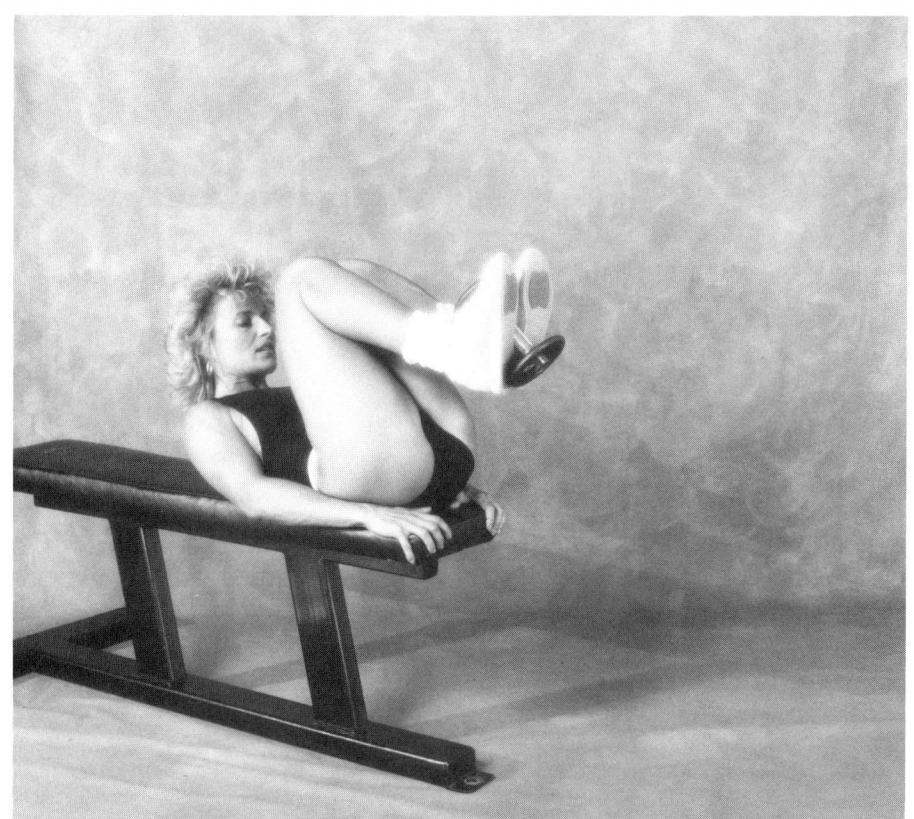

Start

Finish

BUTTOCKS ROUTINE

The buttocks routine requires a special workout. You will not be pyramiding, and you will be doing higher repetitions. The basic formula for the buttocks is three sets of twenty-five repetitions.

All buttocks exercises except the feather kick-up are done with a weight. After a month or two you may find that the weight you are using for an exercise is no longer a challenge. It is time then to increase the weight.

The important thing to remember with buttocks exercises is that the weight is not the primary issue. Weight is there only to provide resistance. Flexing and concentrating are more important.

Some women choose to do their buttocks routine at home before going to the gym since no real gym equipment is necessary to do the buttocks routine. These women also often do their abdominals at home. If you choose to do this, you will save a half hour of gym time.

Feather Kick-up—Buttocks Exercise #1

This exercise develops and lifts the outer areas of the buttocks and helps to eliminate excess fat from that area. It is done without weight. That is why it is called the "feather kick-up."

POSITIONING

- Take an "on all fours" position on a flat exercise bench.
- Raise your right thigh back and bend your knee so that your leg takes the shape of an *L*.

EXERCISE

- Extend your buttocks-to-thigh area as high up as possible until your leg is extended straight upward as high as possible.
- Quickly return to the starting position, and repeat the movement until you have done the correct number of repetitions for your set.
- Do the exercise for the other leg and, alternating right and left, complete the required number of sets for each leg.

ALERT

- You should feel the stress in your upper buttocks (from your waist downward). Flex your buttocks as you perform the movement.
- This exercise is difficult to get used to. Be patient. It's very effective.

"NEVERS"

- Never let your knee lower to the bench. Keep it high and at the *L* position as a return stance. Note the "start" picture. Always return to that position.
- Never cut the movement short. Always try to go as high as you can on the upward movement.

THE GYM WORKOUT 147

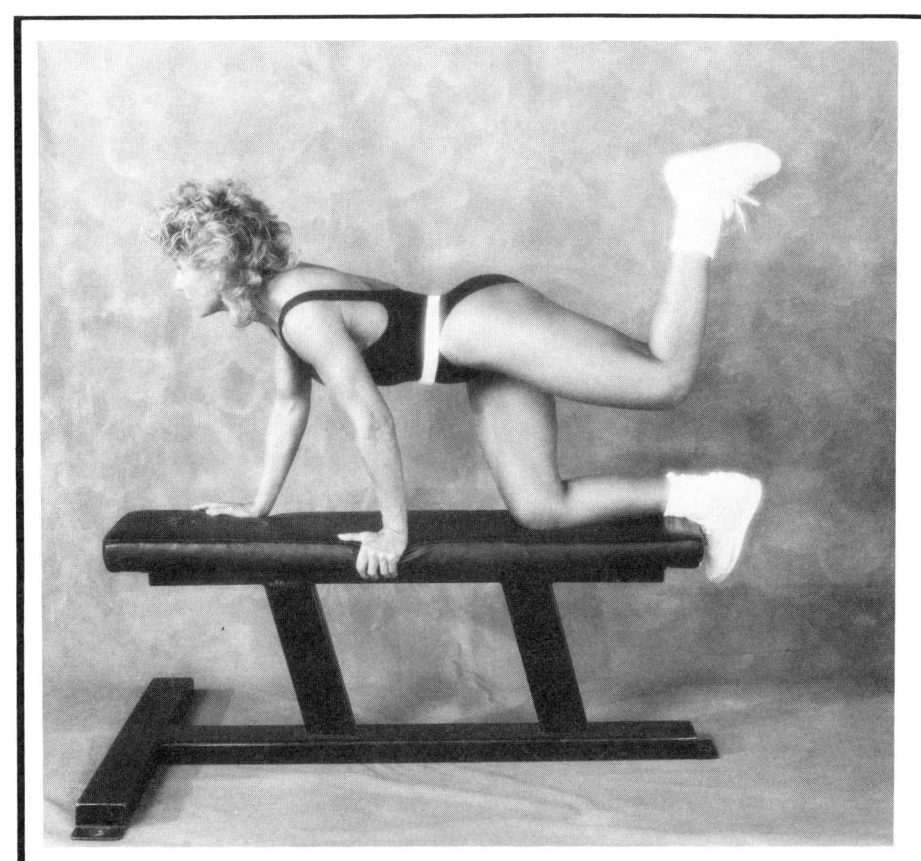

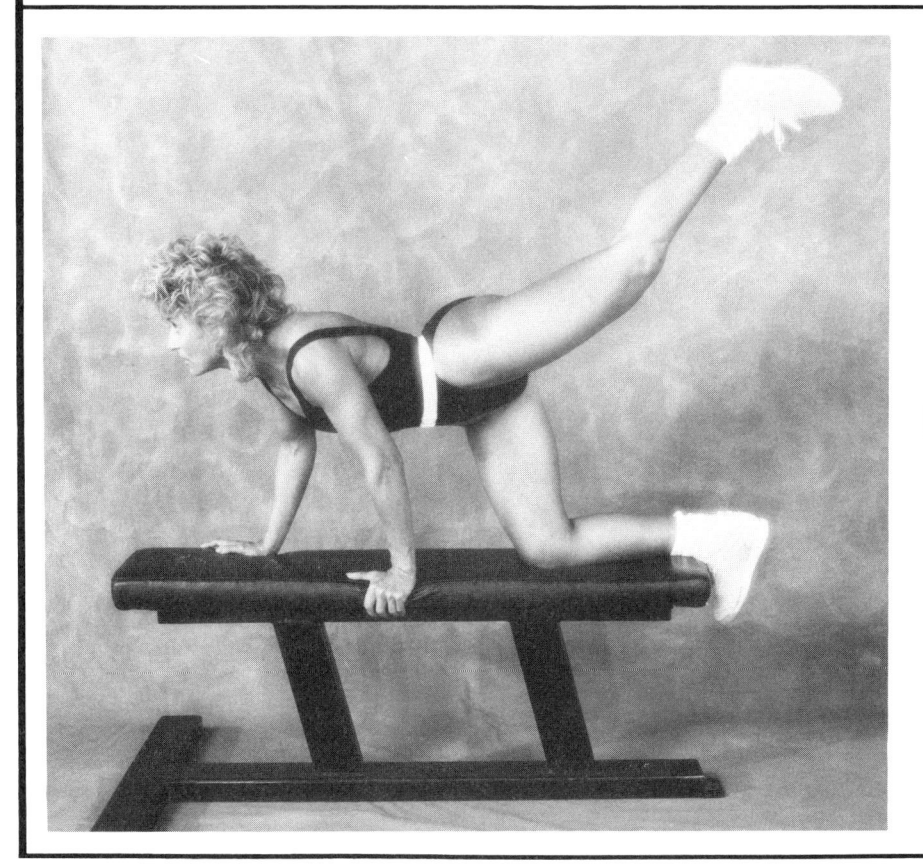

Start

Finish

Scissors—Buttocks Exercise #2

The outer buttock is tightened and excess fat is eliminated by this exercise. The lower buttock is also tightened and "lifted," giving one high rather than sagging buttocks.

POSITIONING

- Place ankle weights on each ankle and seat yourself at the edge of a flat exercise bench.
- Place your hands under your buttocks and extend your legs straight out in front of you. Your buttocks should be close to the end of the bench.
- Bring your legs together for the start position. Your knees should be locked and remain that way for the entire movement.

EXERCISE

- Flexing your buttocks as tightly as possible, spread your legs to the greatest possible extent. Without pausing, return to starting position and repeat the movement until you have performed the correct number of repetitions for your set.

ALERT

- This entire exercise depends upon your flexing your buttock area. As your hands are under the muscles you should be able to feel them flex.
- This exercise can be performed on reverse pulleys using a free-standing pulley machine and ankle straps.

"NEVERS"

- Never cut the movement short. Try to go as wide as possible.
- Never cross your legs over on the return movement. Return your legs to an ankle-touching-ankle position.

THE GYM WORKOUT **149**

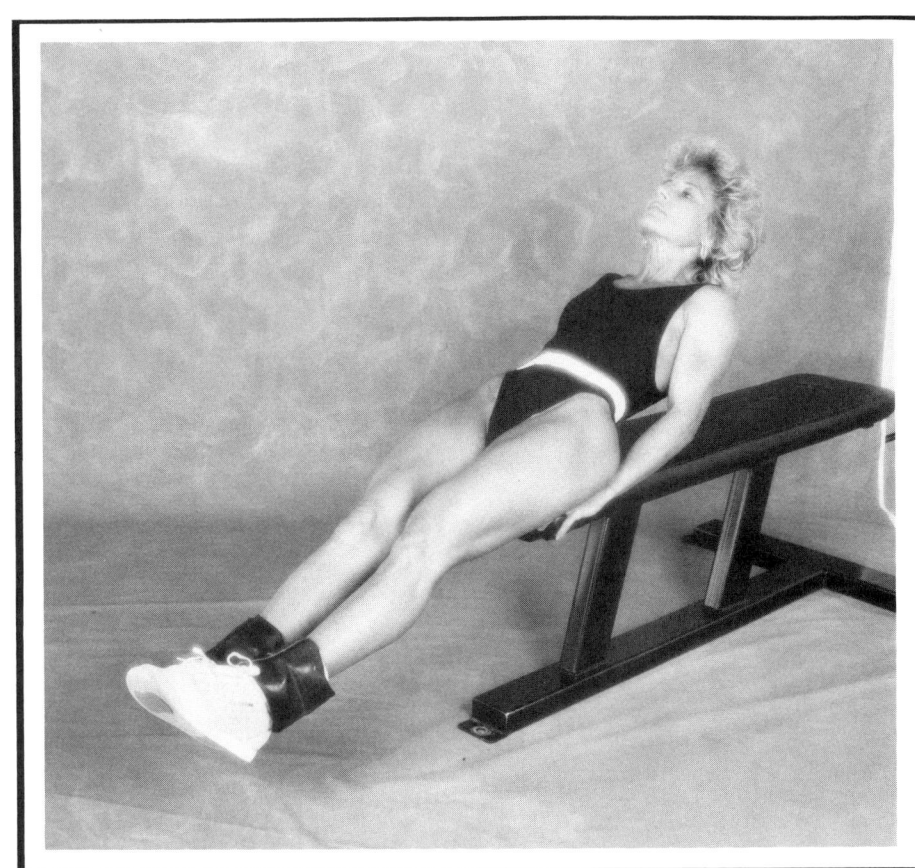

Start

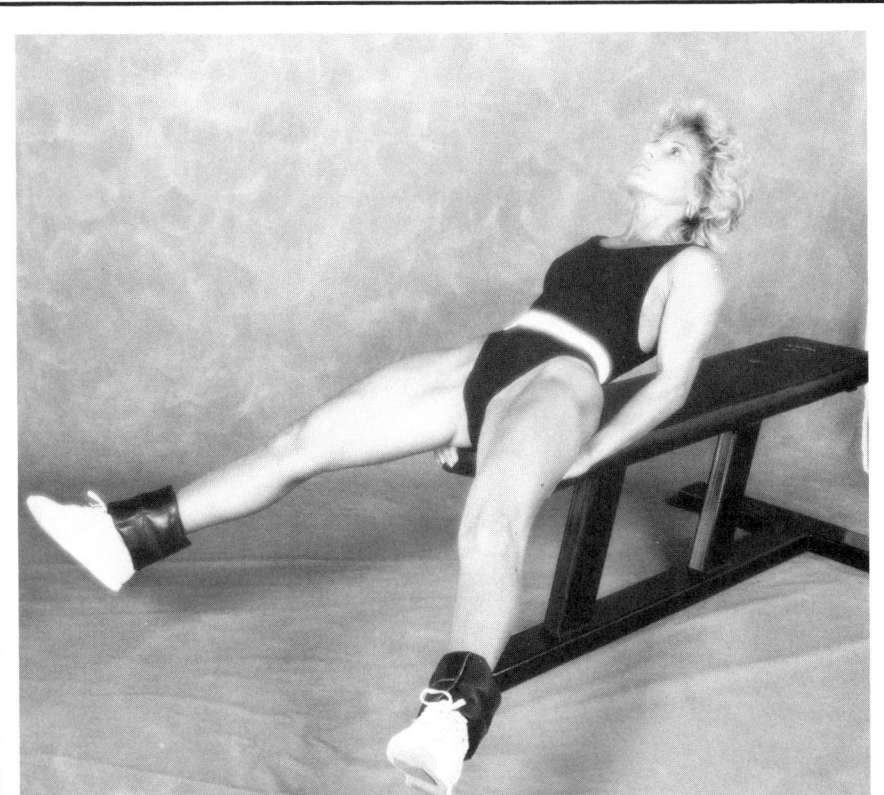

Finish

Back Leg Kick—Buttocks Exercise #3

The buttocks are tightened and lifted; the back thigh (biceps femoris) muscles are also tightened by this exercise.

POSITIONING

- Place the ankle weights or cable attachment around your ankles.
- Lean on a flat exercise bench in an "on all fours" position, but allow your right leg to extend straight down to the floor.
- Stretch your right foot back.

EXERCISE

- Flex your buttocks and, with your knee locked, lift your right leg behind you as high as possible. Keep your toes pointed and your ankle stretched away from you.
- Return to starting position and repeat the movement until you have performed the correct number of repetitions for your set.
- Repeat the set for your left leg. Alternate sets for each leg until you have performed the correct number of sets for the exercise. Do not rest between sets.

ALERT

- As illustrated, this exercise can be performed on the free-standing pulley machine with the use of ankle straps attached to the pulleys. If you choose to use the machine, you will have to switch quickly back and forth as you complete a set for each leg.
- Keep your knee locked and your buttocks flexed throughout the movement.
- Keep your leg moving up in line with your body. Beware of the temptation to let your leg extend out, away from your body.

"NEVERS"

- Never jerk your leg up in an effort to rush through the exercise.
- Never stop flexing your buttocks.

THE GYM WORKOUT **151**

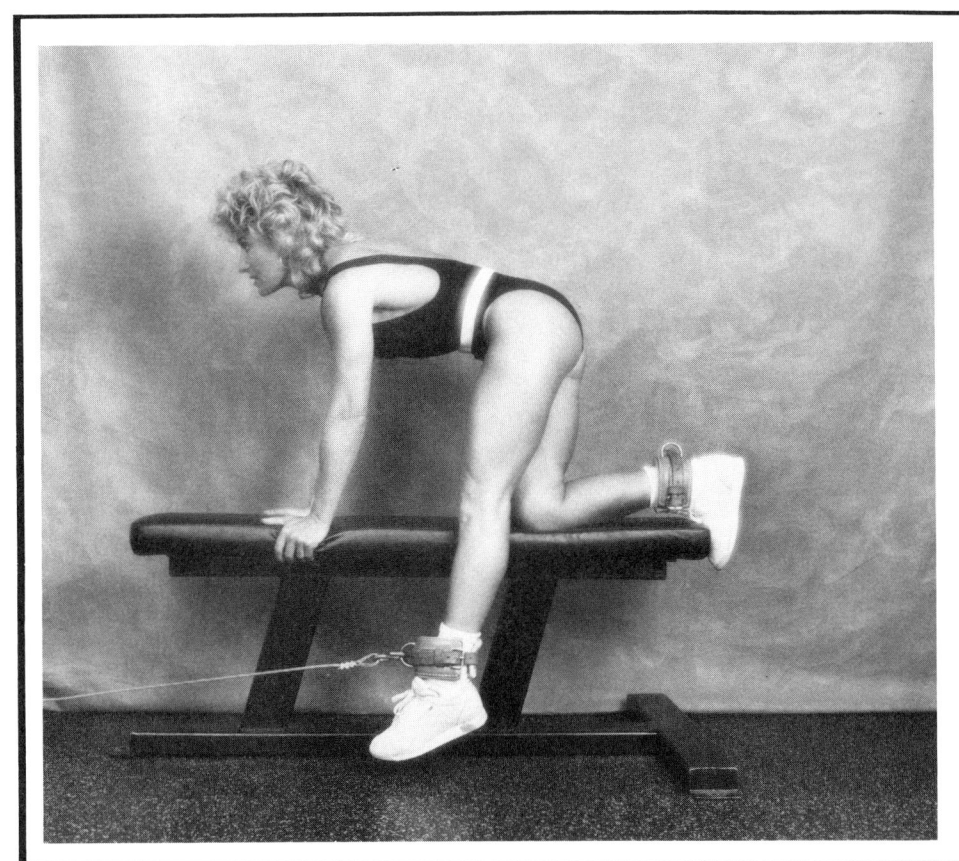

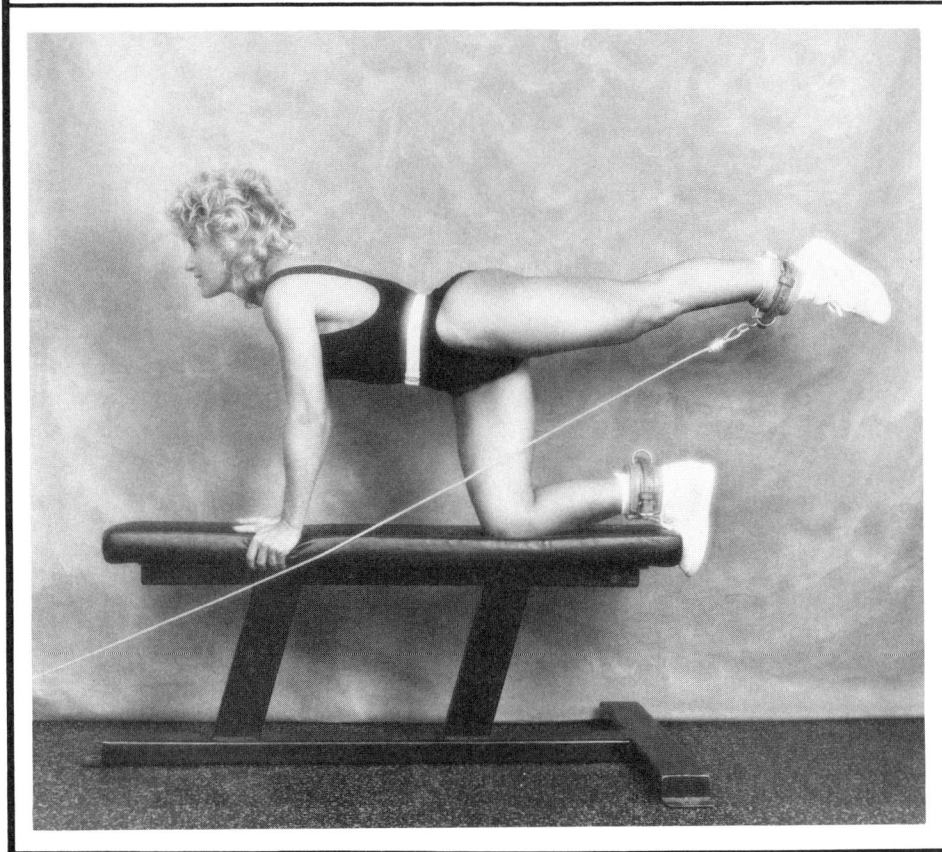

Start

Finish

Barbell Tuck—Buttocks Exercise #4

This exercise tightens and lifts the entire buttocks area and prevents the "sagging butt" look. Success depends on flexing the buttocks hard on each return movement.

POSITIONING

- Stand with your feet a comfortable width apart, with a barbell placed on your shoulders, resting on your trapezius muscles.
- If possible, stand in front of a mirror.

EXERCISE

- Lower yourself five to ten inches, bending at the knee as if you were doing a squat but stopping very short of a full squat. Do not flex yet.
- Raise yourself up, and as you go flex your buttocks as hard as you can. Thrust your pelvic area forward as you "tuck" your buttocks, flexing as hard as you can. Hold this "tuck"-thrust position for a second, then return to the down position.
- Repeat the down-up-tuck movement until you have completed the correct number of repetitions for your set.

ALERT

- The importance of flexing on the tuck movement cannot be overemphasized, as it is the basis of success in this exercise. Feel your buttocks becoming smaller and tighter as you tuck each of the twenty-five times.

"NEVERS"

- Never use a heavy weight for this exercise. Select a comfortable weight. I use forty-five pounds. You may begin with twenty or twenty-five.
- Never let your mind wander during this exercise. Think about what you are doing, and tell your buttocks to take shape.

THE GYM WORKOUT **153**

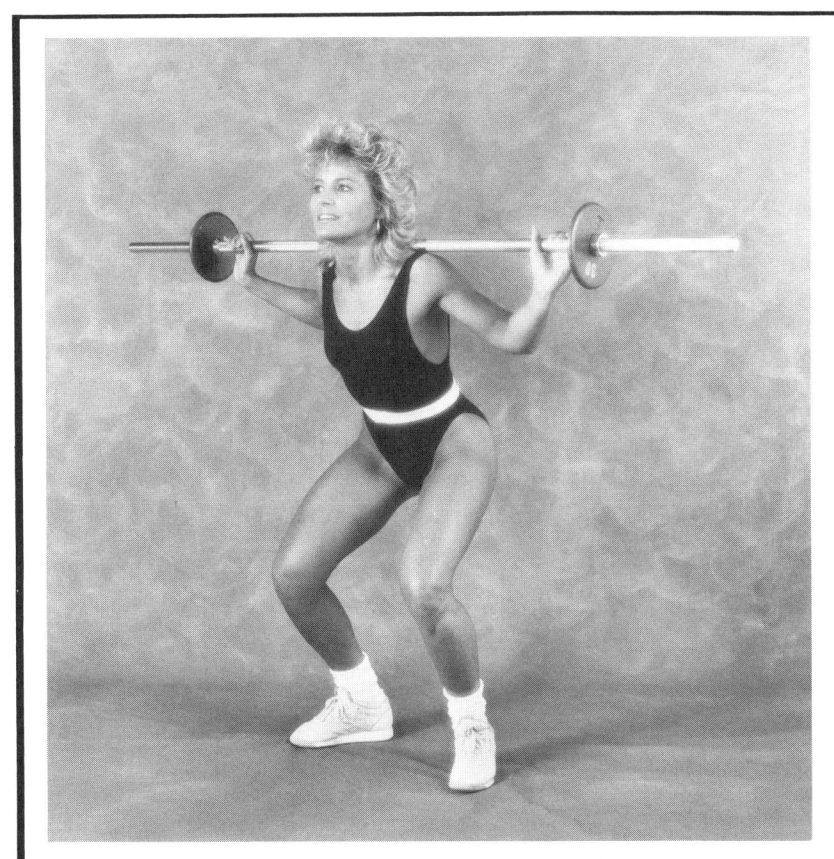

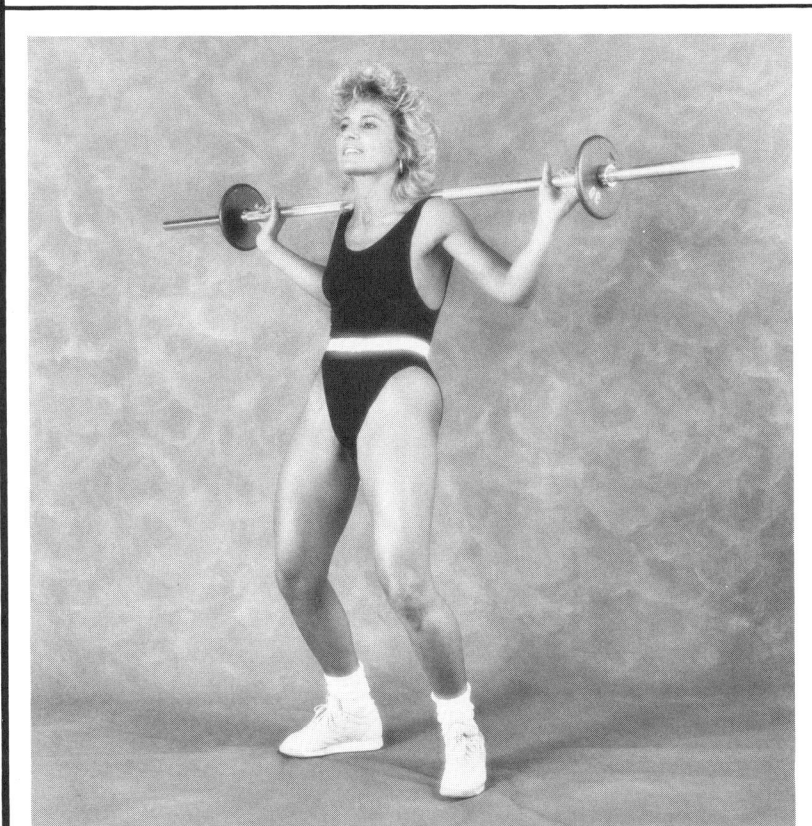

Start

Finish

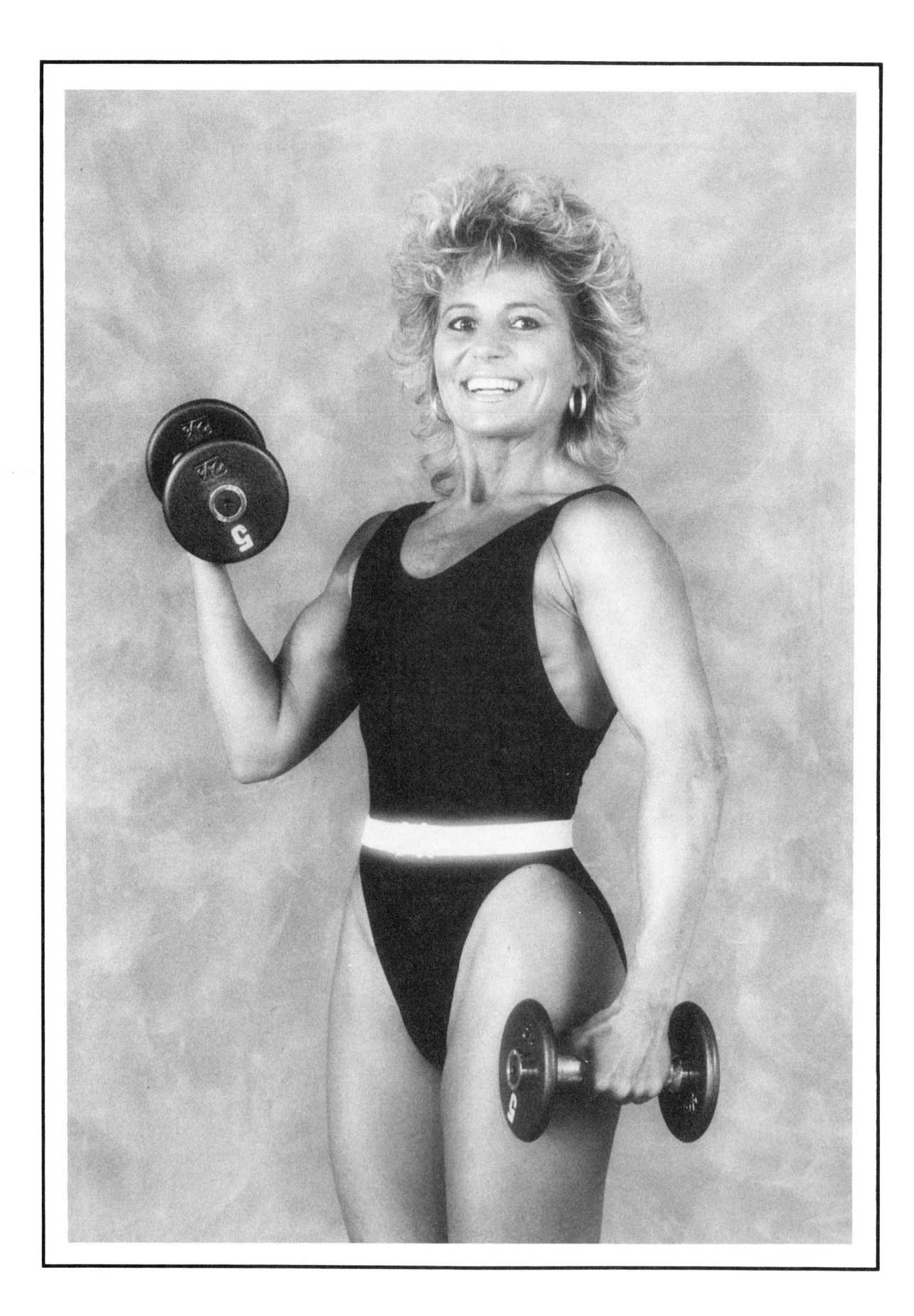

CHAPTER 8

THE HOME WORKOUT

Your home workout will consist of four exercises per body part, three sets per exercise. You will be doing three times four or twelve sets per body part. On training days One and Three you will be doing chest, shoulders, back, abdominals, and buttocks. On training days Two and Four you will be doing biceps, triceps, legs, abdominals, and buttocks.

Review the bodybuilding terms at the beginning of Chapter 5, and Chapter 6, "Preparation for Beginning." Then you will be ready to start your home workout.

DAYS ONE AND THREE

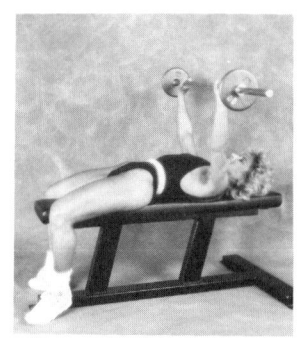

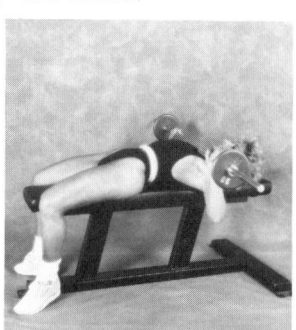

Bench Press— Chest Exercise #1

CHEST ROUTINE

Follow the instructions on page 88. Use a barbell and a free-weight bench press stand.

Incline Flye— Chest Exercise #2

Follow the instructions on page 90.

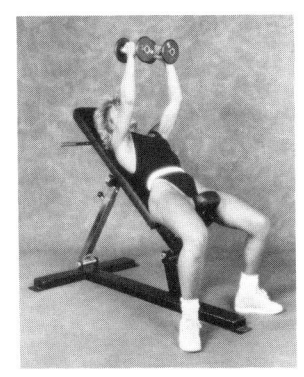

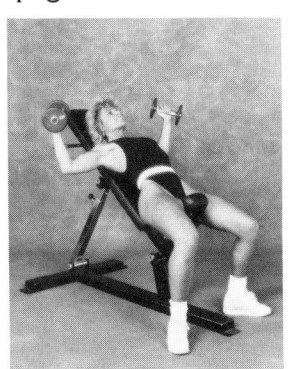

Cross Bench Pullover— Chest Exercise #3

Follow the instructions on page 92. Use a flat exercise bench.

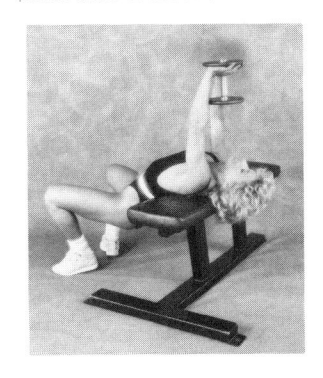

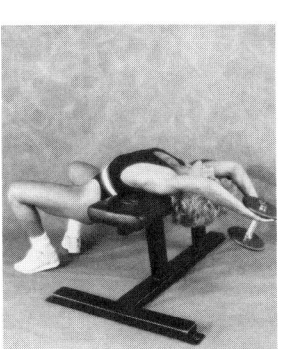

Decline Bench Press—Chest Exercise #4

This exercise stresses the lower pectoral (chest) area and helps lift the muscles there. This exercise is a favorite with women who wish to remedy sagging breasts.

POSITIONING

- Place a block of wood about six to eight inches high at the foot of a flat exercise bench. (You may use a 30° decline bench instead.)
- Lie on the bench with your head toward the lower end and your legs over the elevated end (knees bent and calves extending over the edge of the bench).
- Grasp the barbell with your hands held about two inches wider apart than shoulder width, palms facing outward.
- Lift the barbell straight up to arm's length. You are in starting position.

EXERCISE

- Slowly lower the barbell until it touches your chest. Let your chest muscles stretch out as you perform the movement.
- Raise the barbell to starting position and flex (squeeze together) your pectoral muscles. Repeat the movement until you have performed the correct number of repetitions for your set.

ALERT

- Control the barbell at all times. Picture the muscles growing.

"NEVERS"

- Never rush the movement. Control the barbell and keep it balanced at all times. Flex and stretch. Keep the muscles "working."

THE HOME WORKOUT 159

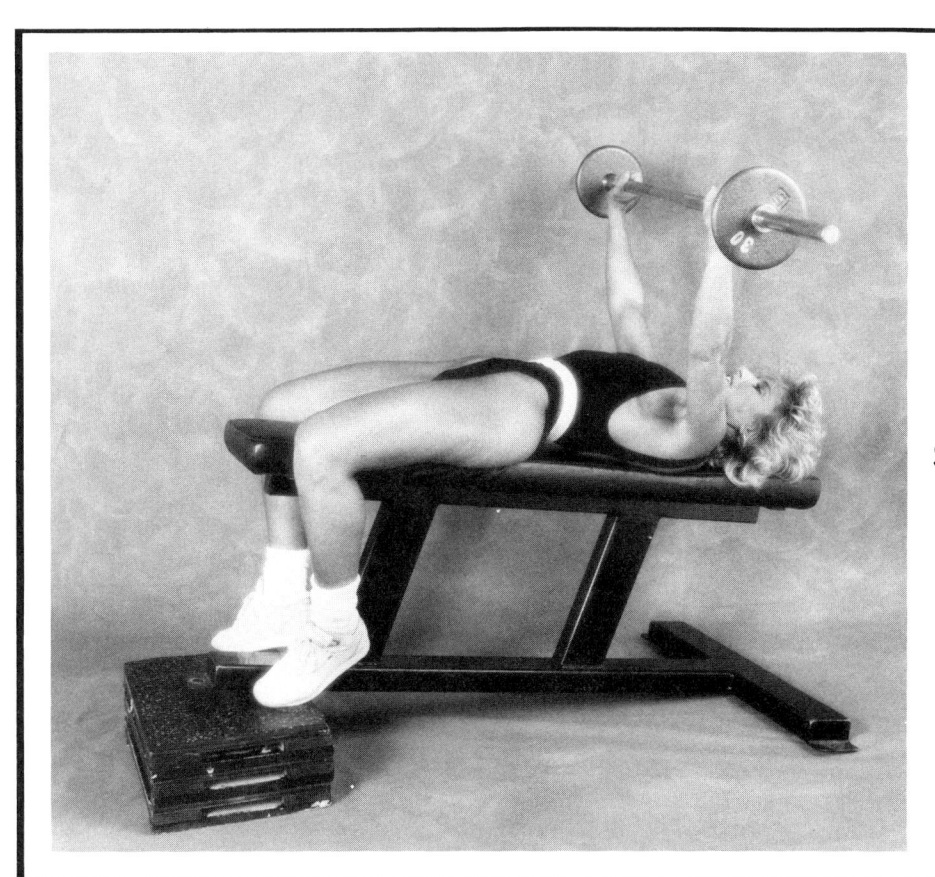

Start

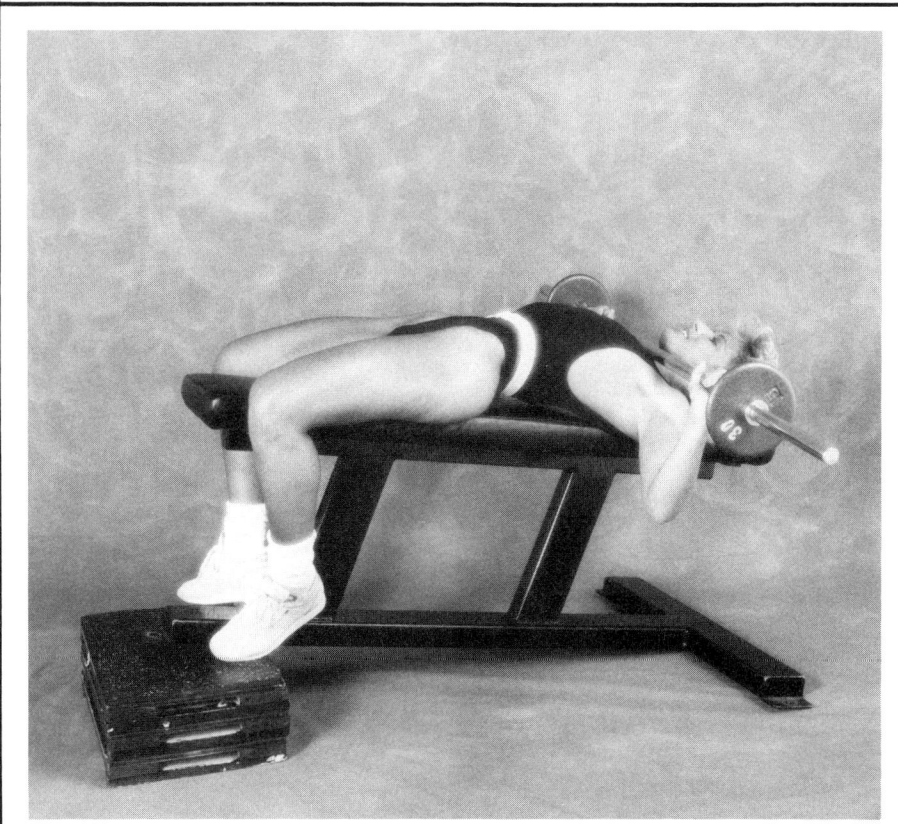

Finish

SHOULDER ROUTINE

Side Lateral Raise— Shoulder Exercise #1

Follow the instructions on page 96.

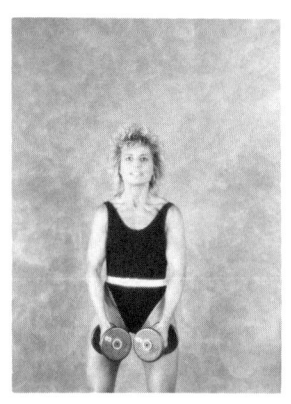

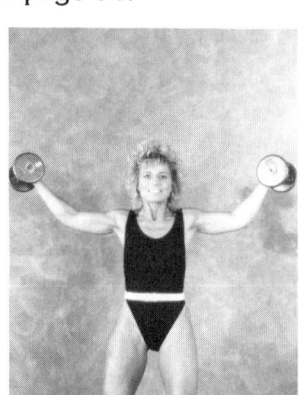

Front Lateral Raise— Shoulder Exercise #2

Follow the instructions on page 98.

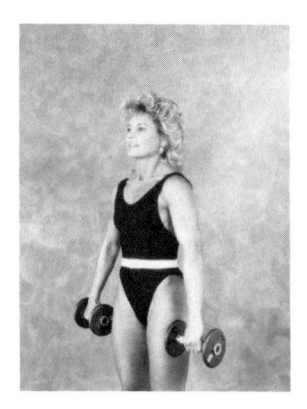

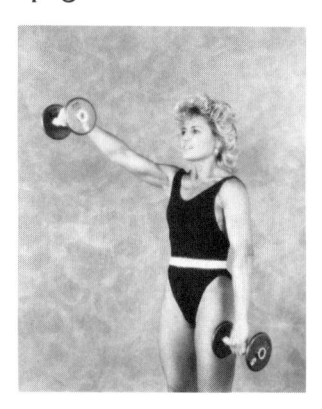

Military Press behind the Neck— Shoulder Exercise #3

Follow the instructions on page 100.

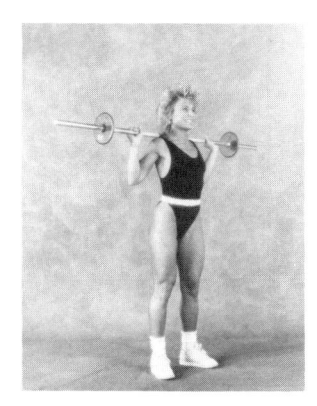

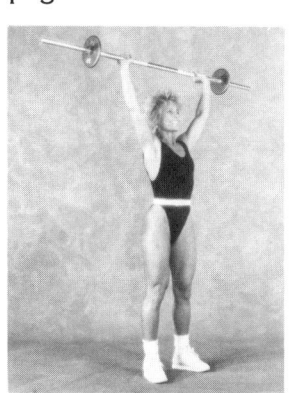

Upright Row— Shoulder Exercise #4

Follow the instructions on page 102.

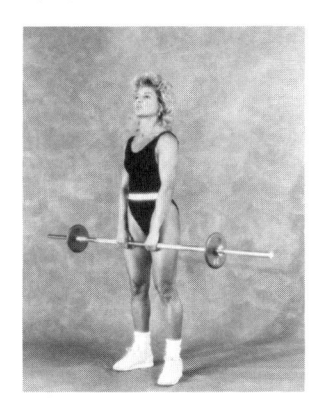

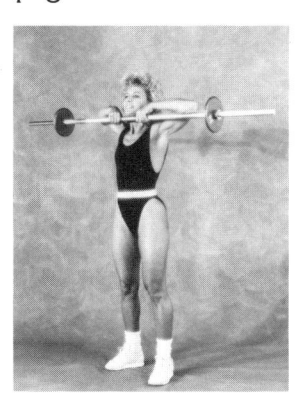

BACK ROUTINE

This exercise develops the latissimus dorsi, or "lat," muscles of your back.

Spinal Lifts—Back Exercise #1

POSITIONING

- Lie on a mat on the floor, flat on your stomach.
- Extend your arms straight out in front of you and grasp a broomstick or other stick in your hands, palms facing the floor. Your grip should be about three inches wider than shoulder width.

EXERCISE

- Grasping the stick, raise your arms and your legs at the same time, never letting your abdominal area leave the mat.
- Go as high as you can, concentrating on raising both upper and lower body at the same time. Be sure that your knees are locked. You should feel the stretch in your back.
- Repeat the movement until you have completed the correct number of repetitions for your set.

ALERT

- Concentrate on moving the lower and upper body together in an effort to form an arch. Imagine that you are trying to touch your feet and the stick together at the center of your back.

"NEVERS"

- Never jerk yourself up in an effort to get higher. You could pull your back.
- Never rest on the down position until you have completed a full set.

One-Arm Dumbbell Bent Row—Back Exercise #2

Follow the instructions on page 108.

THE HOME WORKOUT **163**

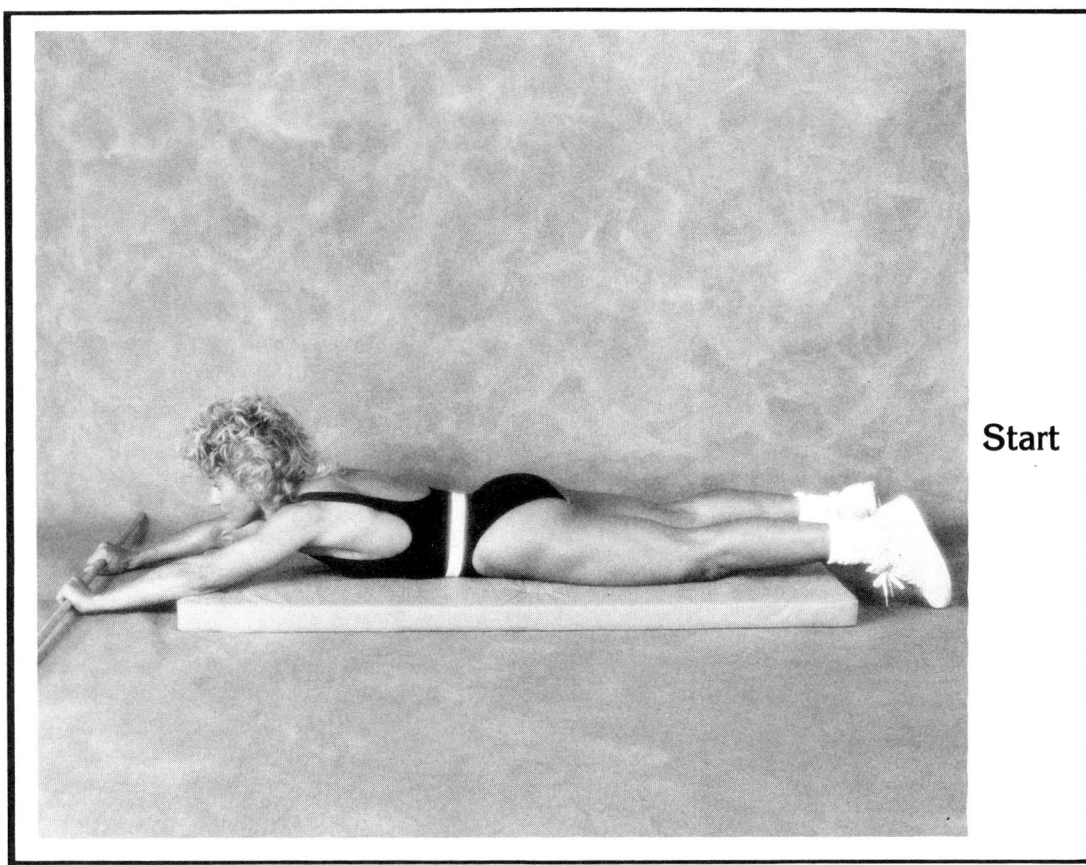

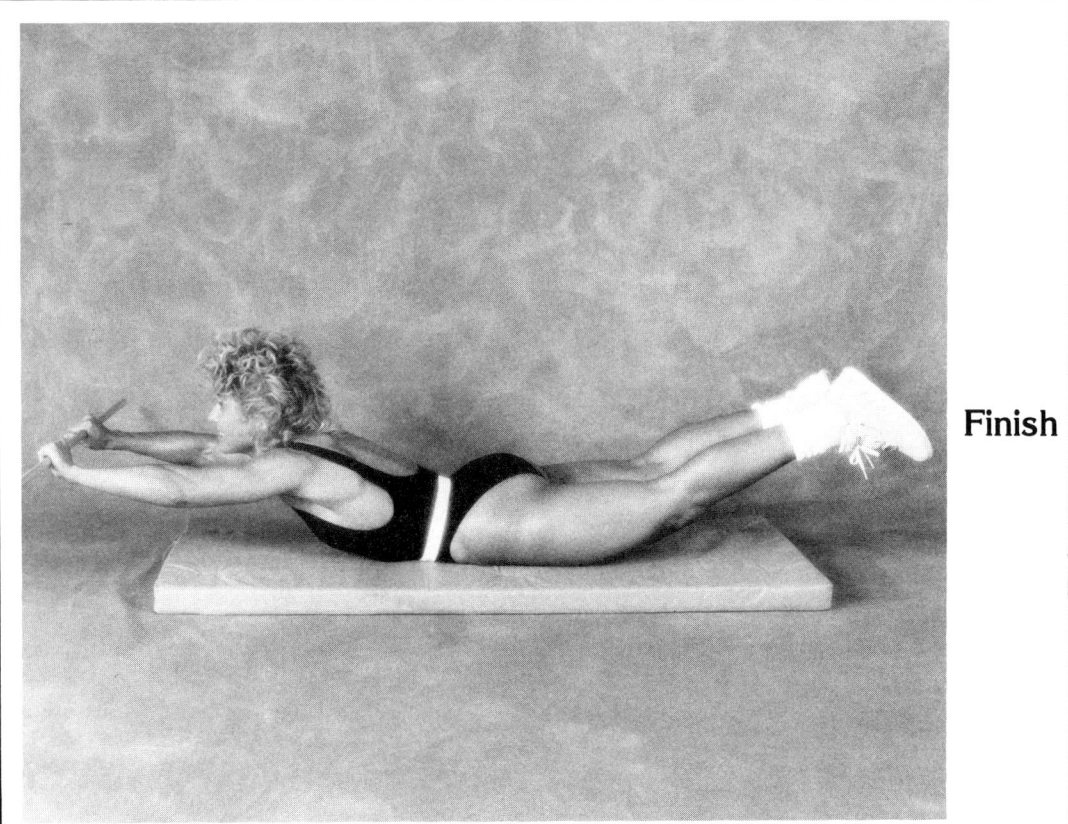

Start

Finish

Seated Dumbbell Rear Laterals—Back Exercise #3

This exercise develops the rear deltoids (shoulders) and slightly stresses the trapezius muscles.

POSITIONING

- Sit at the edge of a flat exercise bench with your buttocks just enough on the bench to keep you from falling off.
- Hold a light dumbbell in each hand, palms facing your body.
- Your feet should be flat on the floor.
- Lean forward until your torso almost touches your thighs, and bring the dumbbells together under your legs until they are almost touching.

EXERCISE

- Slowly extend your arms outward in an arc until they are almost in line with your shoulders. Squeeze your shoulder blades together as you do this. Your torso and head will lift a few inches as you arrive at the finish position.
- Return to start, maintaining control of the weight, and repeat the movement until you have performed the correct number of repetitions for your set.

ALERT

- This is a difficult exercise to get used to, and cheating is common. Study the pictures, and be sure to follow the instructions exactly. You will have to use a very light weight in the beginning in order to do the exercise in strict form.
- Remember to flex (squeeze your shoulder blades together) on the finish position.

"NEVERS"

- Never let the dumbbells just drop into the start position. Control them at all times.
- Never start doing the work with your shoulders by sitting up in a perpendicular position on the up movement.
- Never yield to the temptation to lurch the weights into finish position. Concentrate and maintain control at all times.

THE HOME WORKOUT **165**

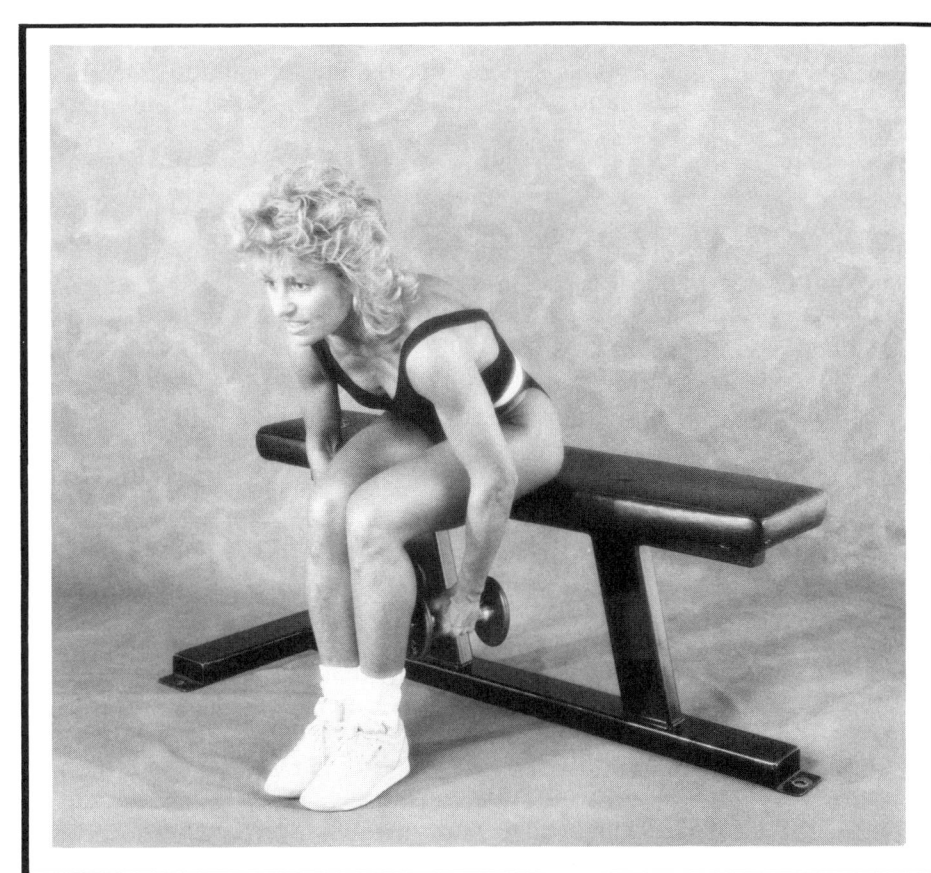

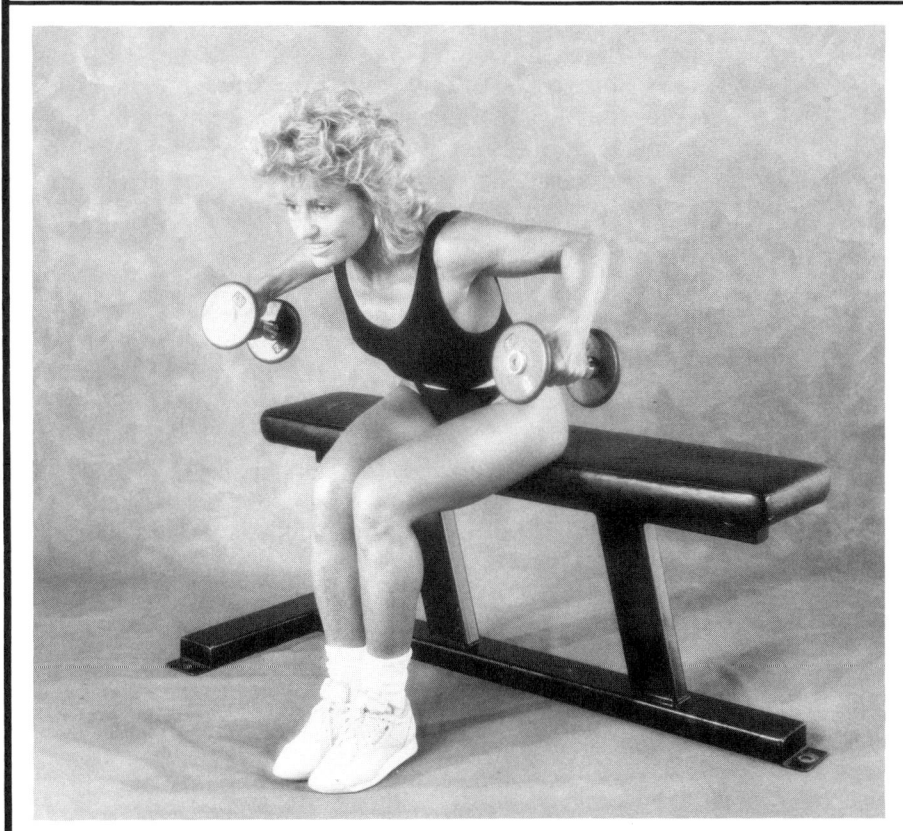

Start

Finish

Bent-Knee Deadlifts— Back Exercise #4

This exercise develops the upper back muscle, the latissimus dorsi, or "lat," muscles, and the trapezius muscles.

POSITIONING

- Place a barbell in front of you on the floor, and stand with feet shoulder width apart.
- Grasp the barbell with hands shoulder width apart, palms facing your body.
- Bend your knees in a ready position.

EXERCISE

- Slowly lift the barbell by rising from the hips, keeping your head up and your back straight.
- Continue to rise with the barbell until you are standing straight, and raise your shoulders up and back, flexing (squeezing) them together. Your arms should be straight down, elbows locked, with the barbell resting against your thighs.
- Hold the flexed position for a split second, then return to starting position. Repeat the movement until you have performed the correct number of repetitions for your set.

ALERT

- Remember to pull your shoulders back as far as possible and to keep your arms straight at your sides and elbows locked on the up position.
- Remember to bend your knees in the start position and to lock your knees in the finish position.

"NEVERS"

- Never jerk the weight into position on the upward movement. Instead, move into position fluidly.
- Never let the weight simply drop to the starting position in an effort to escape the weight. Control the barbell at all times, lowering it slowly and evenly.

Do your Abdominal and Buttocks Routines now. See pages 182–185.

THE HOME WORKOUT 167

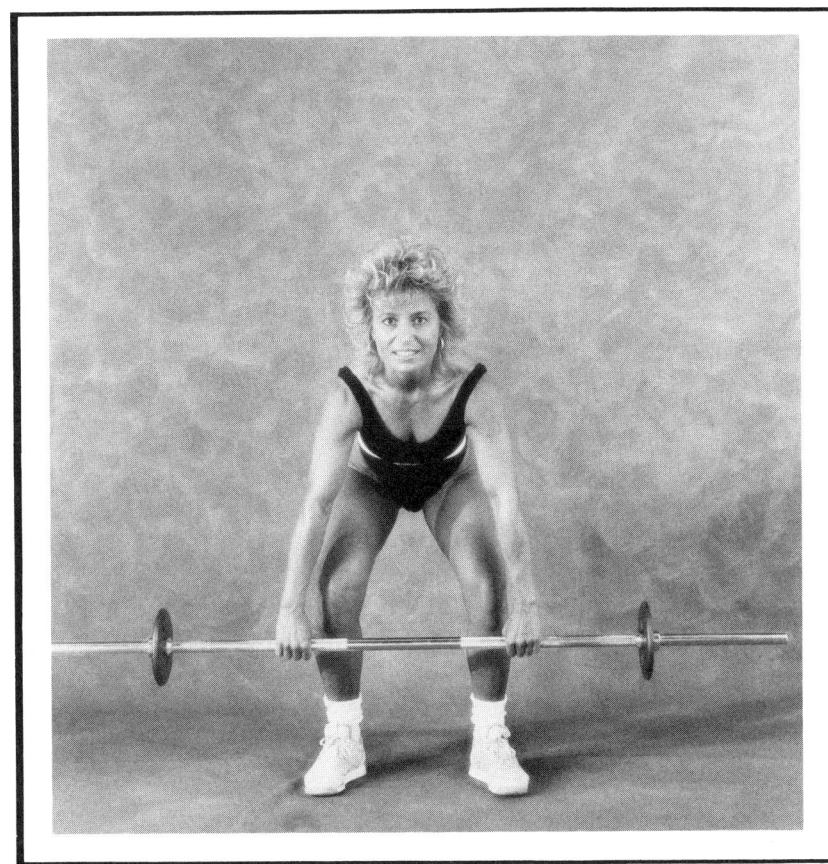

Start

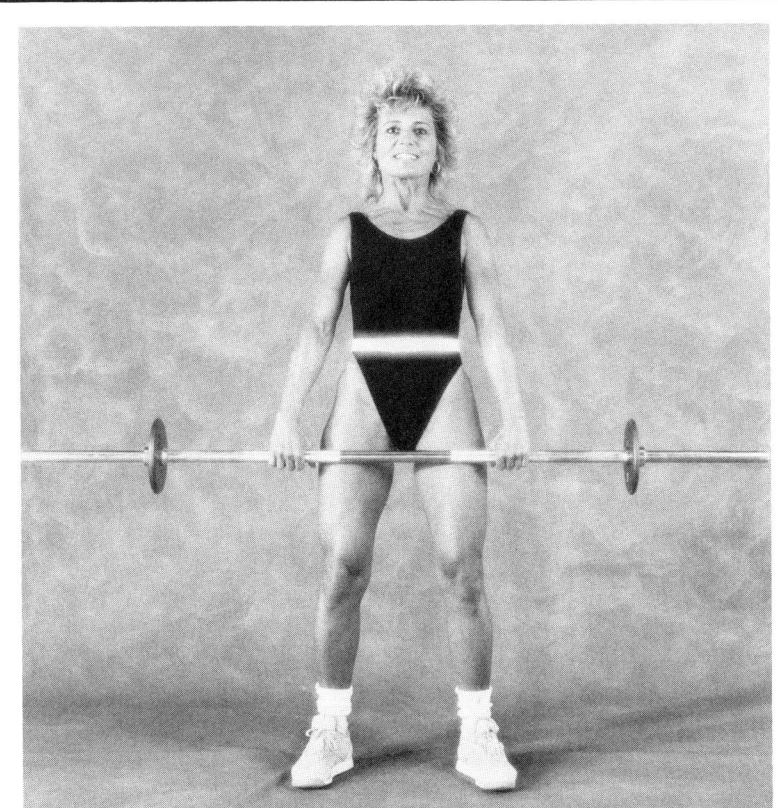

Finish

168 NOW OR NEVER

DAYS TWO AND FOUR

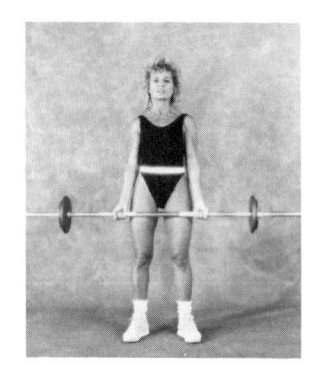

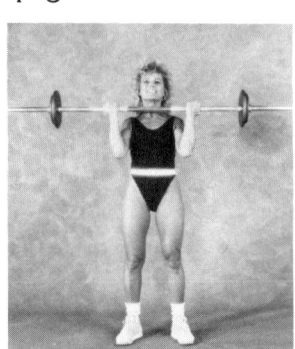

Standing Barbell Curl— Biceps Exercise #1

BICEPS ROUTINE

Follow the instructions on page 112.

THE HOME WORKOUT 169

Concentration
Curl—
Biceps Exercise
#2

Follow the instructions on page 116.

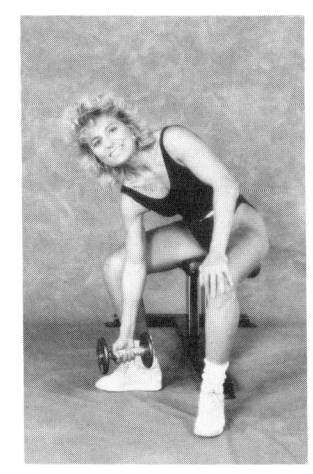

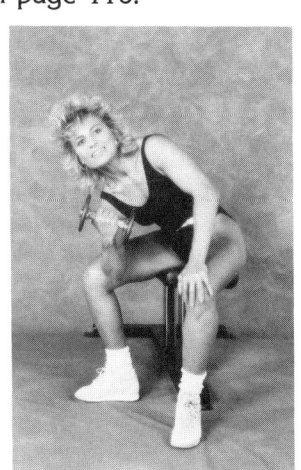

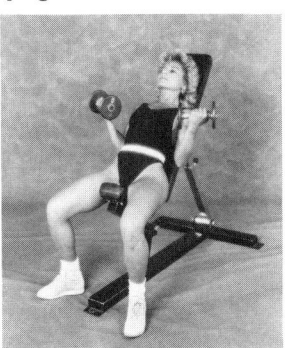

Incline
Dumbbell Curl—
Biceps Exercise
#3

Follow the instructions on page 118.

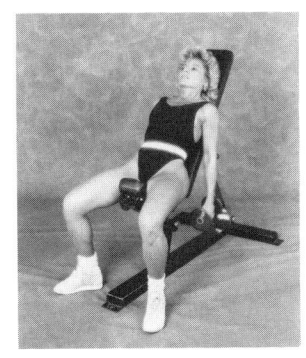

Standing Alternating Dumbbell Curl—Biceps Exercise #4

The entire biceps area is developed by this exercise.

POSITIONING

- Stand with your feet a natural width apart and take one dumbbell in each hand, palms facing your sides.
- Let your arms fall straight down at your sides.

EXERCISE

- Keeping your upper arm close to your side at all times, raise the dumbbell in your right hand to shoulder height, turning your palm upward as you lift. Your elbow should be touching your waist.
- As you lower your right arm to starting position, begin raising the dumbbell in your left hand to shoulder height. Remember to turn your left palm upward as you did with your right palm.
- Repeat the alternating arm movement until you have completed the correct number of repetitions for your set.

ALERT

- If possible, look at yourself in the mirror as you perform this exercise, observing your biceps muscle as it bulges on the flex and stretches out on the downward movement.
- Flex as hard as possible on the upward movement.

"NEVERS"

- Never allow your body to sway in an effort to give momentum to your arm movement. Hold your body erect and steady.
- Never let the dumbbells simply drop to starting position. Maintain control at all times, lowering them slowly and evenly.

THE HOME WORKOUT **171**

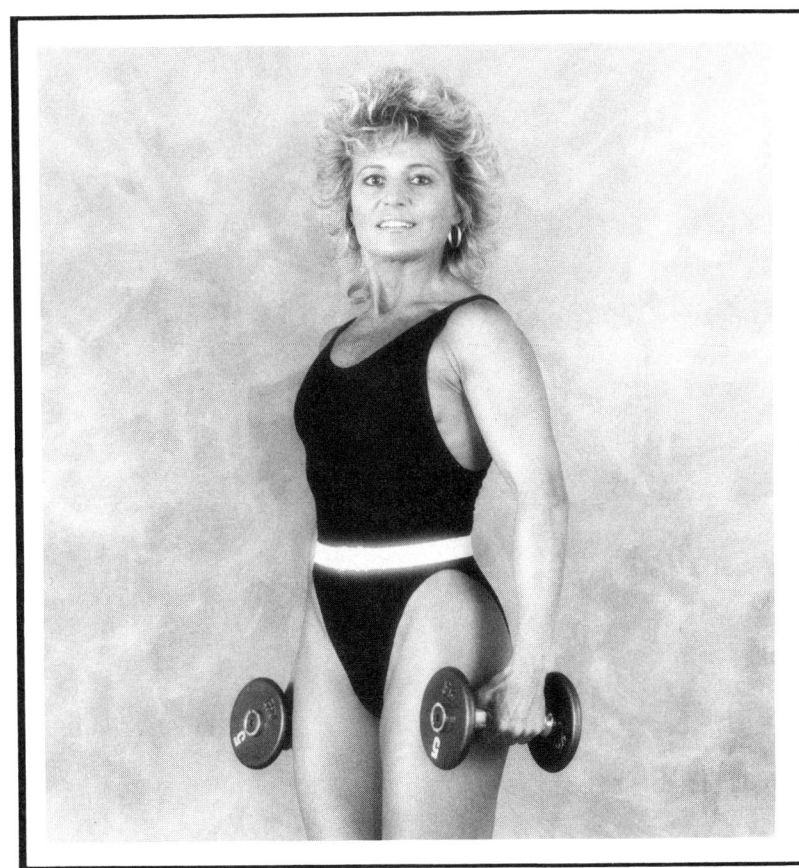

Start

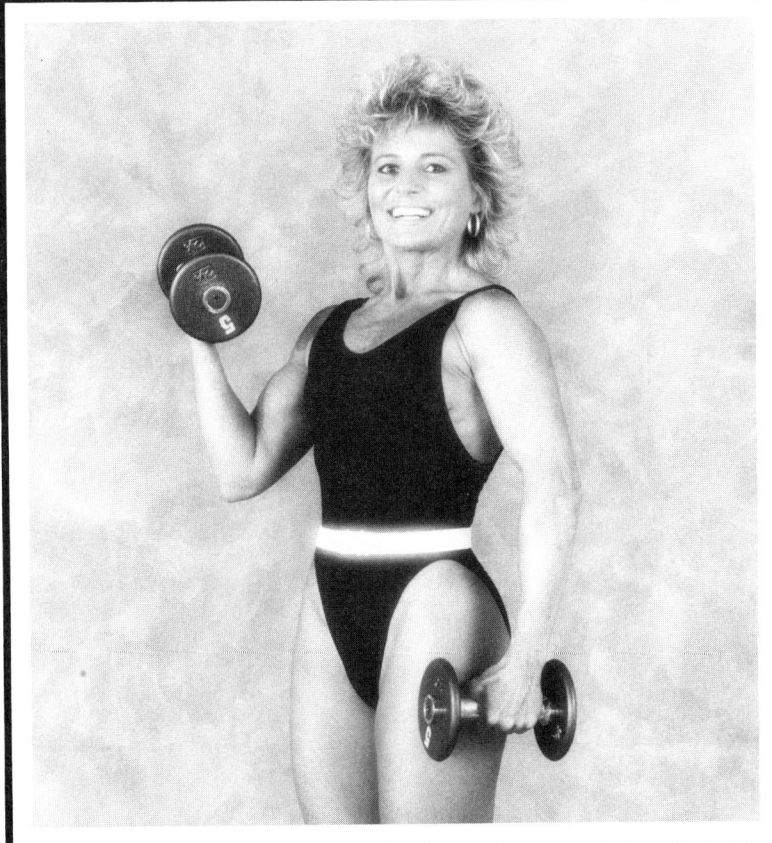

Finish

TRICEPS ROUTINE

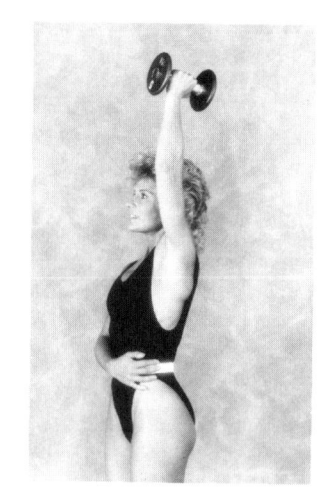

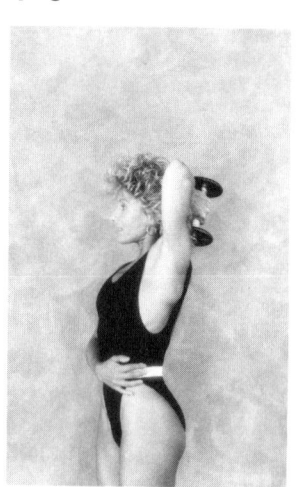

One-Arm Dumbbell Triceps Extension— Triceps Exercise #1

Follow the instructions on page 120.

THE HOME WORKOUT 173

Lying Triceps Extension— Triceps Exercise #2

Follow the instructions on page 122.

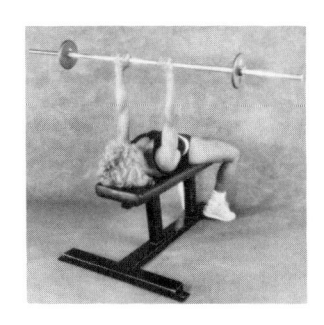

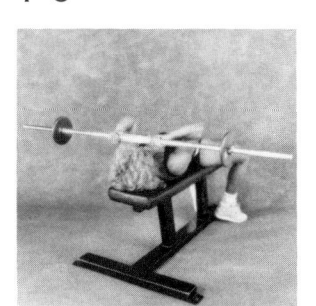

Dips between Benches— Triceps Exercise #3

Follow the instructions on page 126.

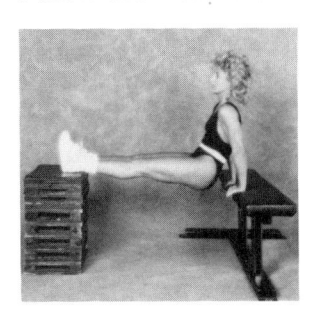

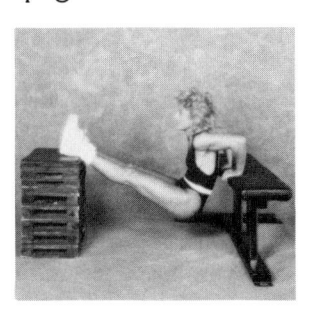

Dumbbell Kickback—Triceps Exercise #4

The entire triceps area is developed by this exercise, preventing the "hanging triceps" look.

POSITIONING

- Holding a dumbbell in your right hand, place your left hand on a flat exercise bench, bending at the waist so that your torso is parallel to the floor.
- Hold your (right) upper arm tight against your body and your elbow tight to your waist.

EXERCISE

- Leaning on the bench with your left arm for support (the left arm is bent), slowly extend your right arm with the dumbbell out behind you, making sure to keep your elbow pinned to your waist. Flex your triceps as your arm reaches full extension.
- Return to starting position and repeat the movement until you have performed the correct number of repetitions for your set.
- Repeat the exercise for the other arm. Alternate arms until you have performed the correct number of sets for the exercise. Do not rest between sets since each arm has a rest while the other works.

ALERT

- Your elbow should act as a hinge for your wrist-to-elbow area.
- Keep your mind on your triceps muscle. Flex. Concentrate.

"NEVERS"

- Never let your elbow pull away from your body.
- Never swing the dumbbell out in an effort to rush the exercise.

THE HOME WORKOUT 175

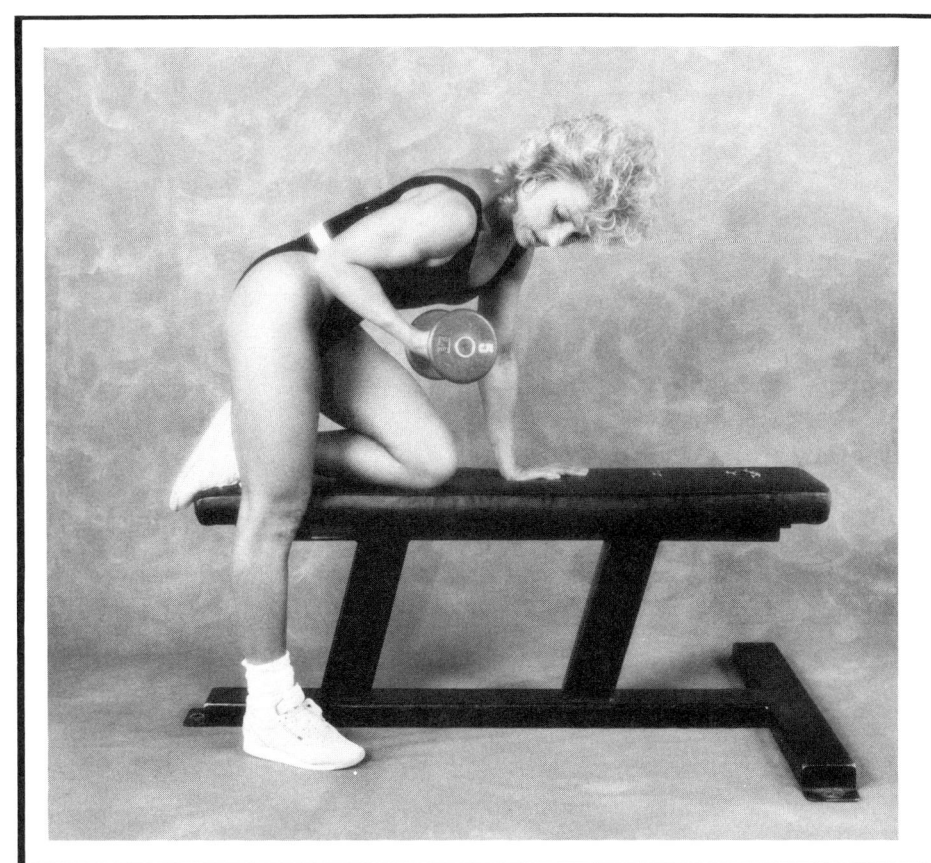

Start

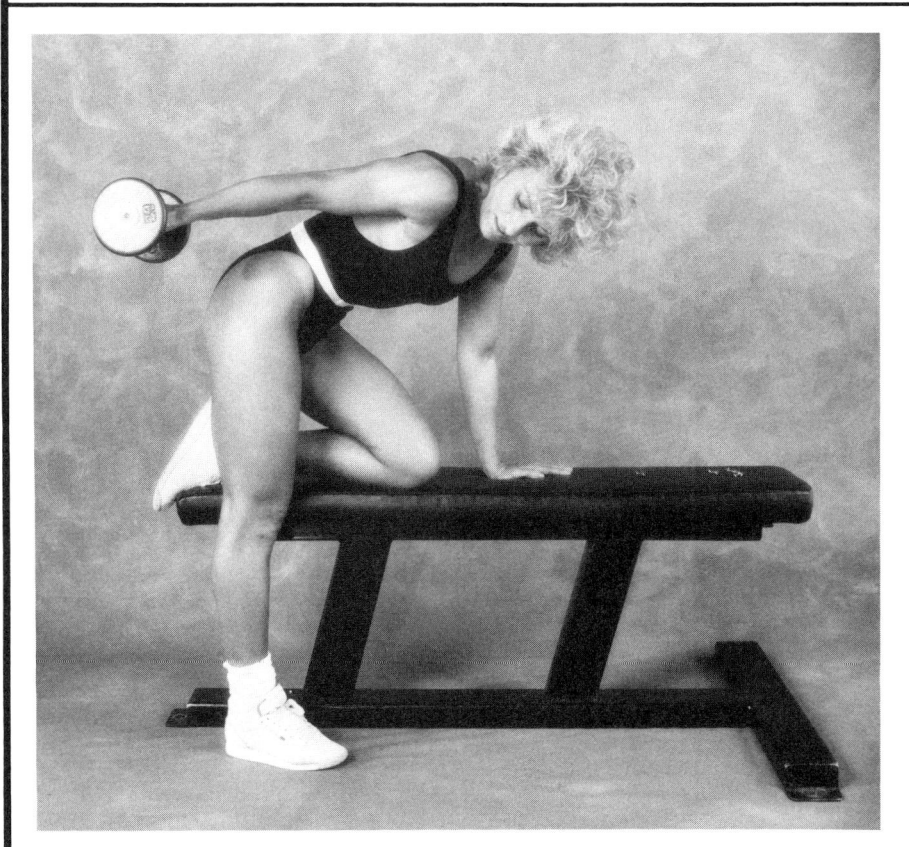

Finish

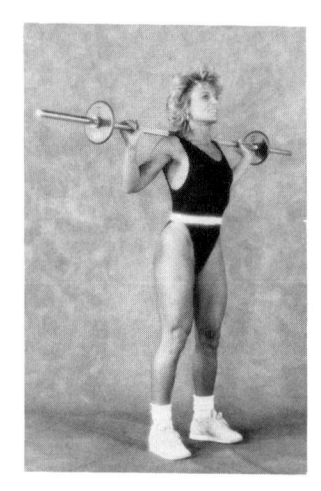

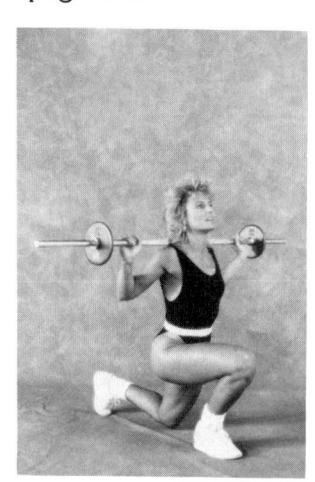

Lunge—
Leg Exercise
#1

LEG ROUTINE

Follow the instructions on page 128.

THE HOME WORKOUT 177

Squat—
Leg Exercise
#2

Follow the instructions on page 130.

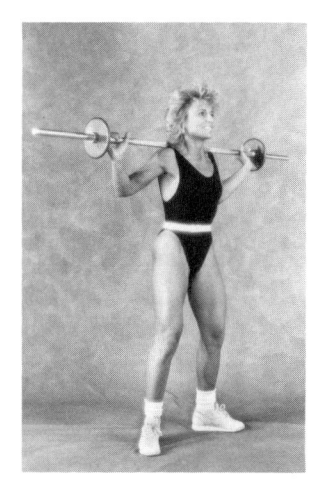

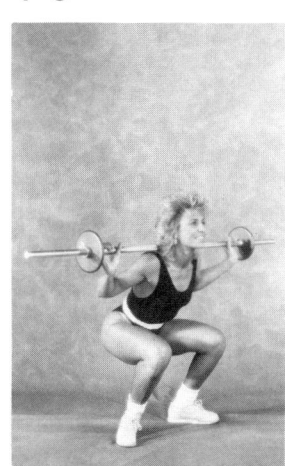

Standing Leg Extension— Leg Exercise #3

The front thigh (quadriceps) is developed by this exercise. Do it without a weight for the first three weeks, and add a two-pound ankle weight after that. You may go as high as five pounds for each ankle, in time.

POSITIONING

- Stand with your feet a natural width apart.
- Let your arms hang naturally at your sides.

EXERCISE

- Raise your right thigh perpendicular to your body, with your knee bent at a right angle.
- Extend your leg straight out, locking your knee and flexing your thigh (quadriceps) muscle. Your fully extended leg should be parallel to the floor. Keep your thigh flexed for two seconds.
- Return to the right angle position, and stretch your quadriceps muscle, then return to starting position.
- Repeat the four-step movement until you have performed the correct number of repetitions for your set.
- Repeat the exercise for the left leg. Then return to the right leg and continue to alternate legs until you have performed the correct number of sets for the exercise.

ALERT

- Be sure to flex, and watch the quadriceps muscle as it bulges on the flex.

"NEVERS"

- Never rush the exercise.
- Never forget to do each repetition in a sequence of four distinct steps, holding a moment between each step.

THE HOME WORKOUT **179**

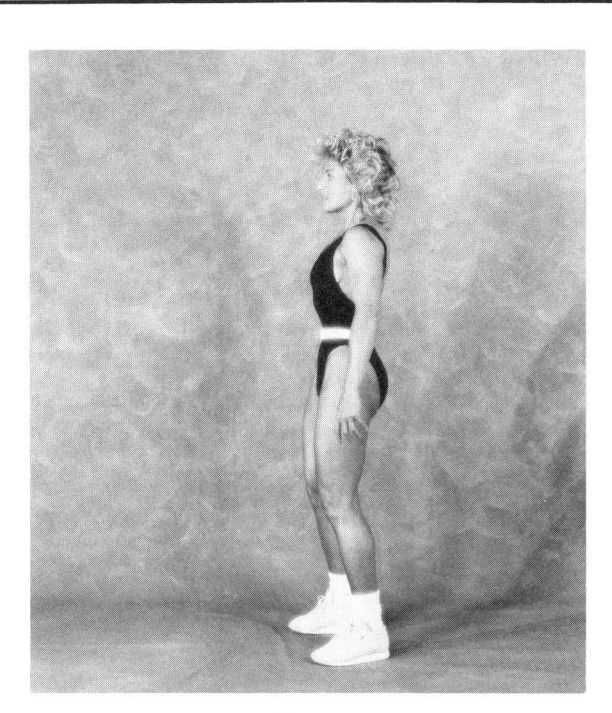

Start

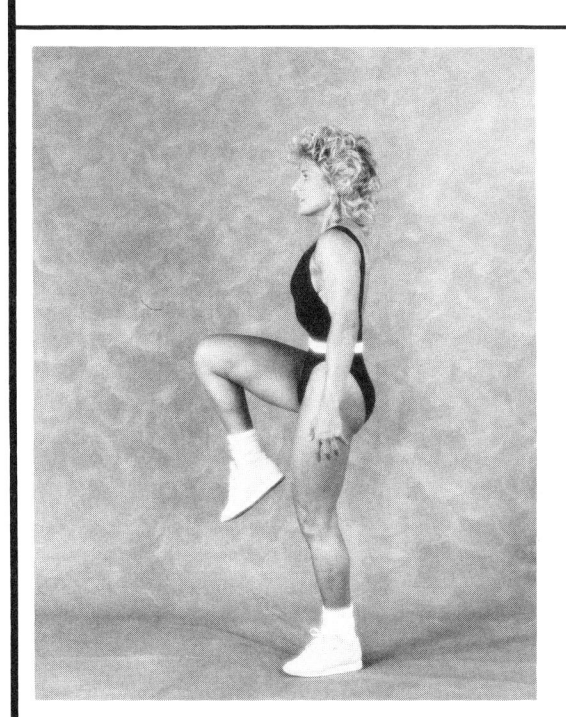

Midpoint

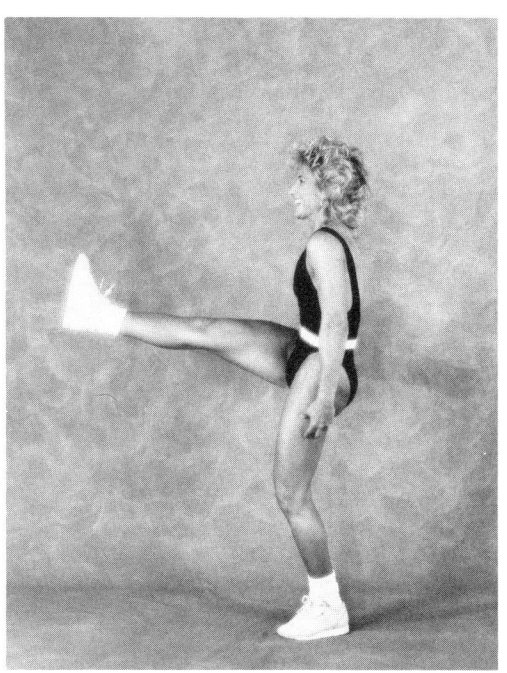

Finish

Dumbbell Leg Curl—Leg Exercise #4

The back thigh (biceps femoris, or hamstring) muscles are developed by this exercise. It can be performed lying either on a flat exercise bench or a table.

POSITIONING

- Lie facedown on the exercise bench or table with your knees touching its lower edge.
- Place a small dumbbell between your feet, positioning it so that you can hold it with the arches of your feet.

EXERCISE

- Slowly bend your legs at the knee, raising your feet upward until your lower legs are perpendicular to the floor. Your legs should be at a 90° angle. Flex your back thigh muscles.
- Maintaining your grip on the weight, slowly return to starting position and repeat the movement until you have performed the correct number of repetitions for your set.

ALERT

- Concentrate on your back thigh muscles as you do the exercise. Picture the cellulite wearing away and firm muscles forming.

"NEVERS"

- Never arch your back up from the bench or table. Keep your abdominal area glued to the surface.
- Never swing the weight up hurriedly. It may fly loose and hit you in the head.
- Never let your legs just drop into start position of themselves. Work hard to control the weight throughout the movement, feeling the muscle work as it stretches and flexes.

One-Leg Toe Raise—Leg Exercise #5

Follow the instructions on page 136.

THE HOME WORKOUT 181

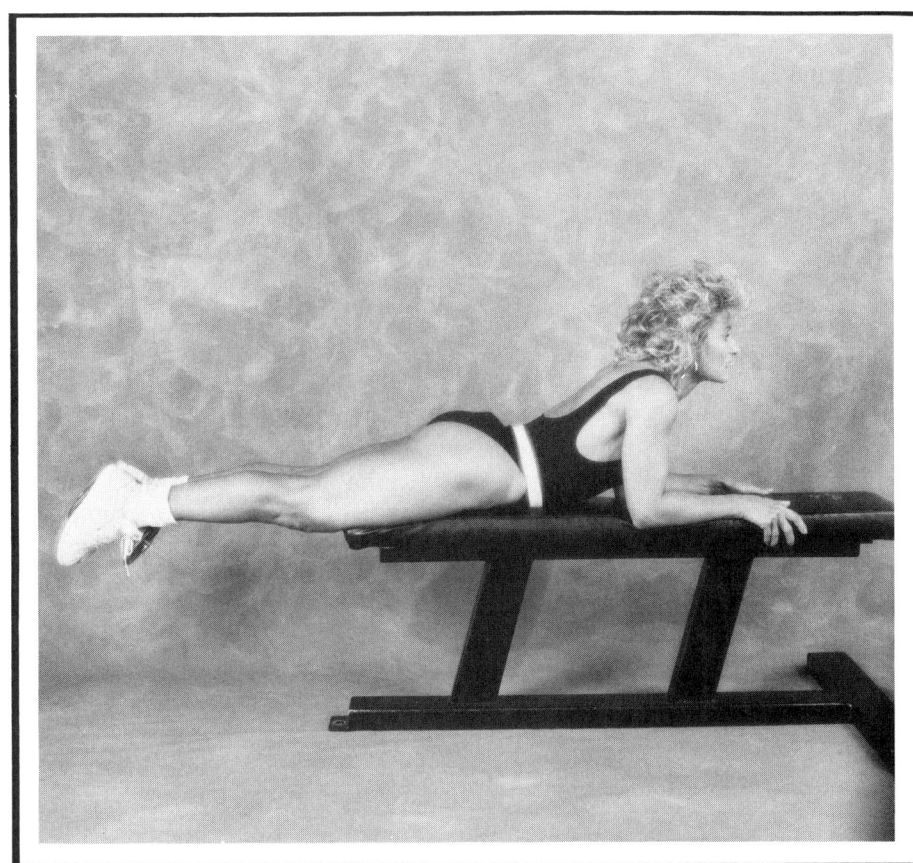

Start

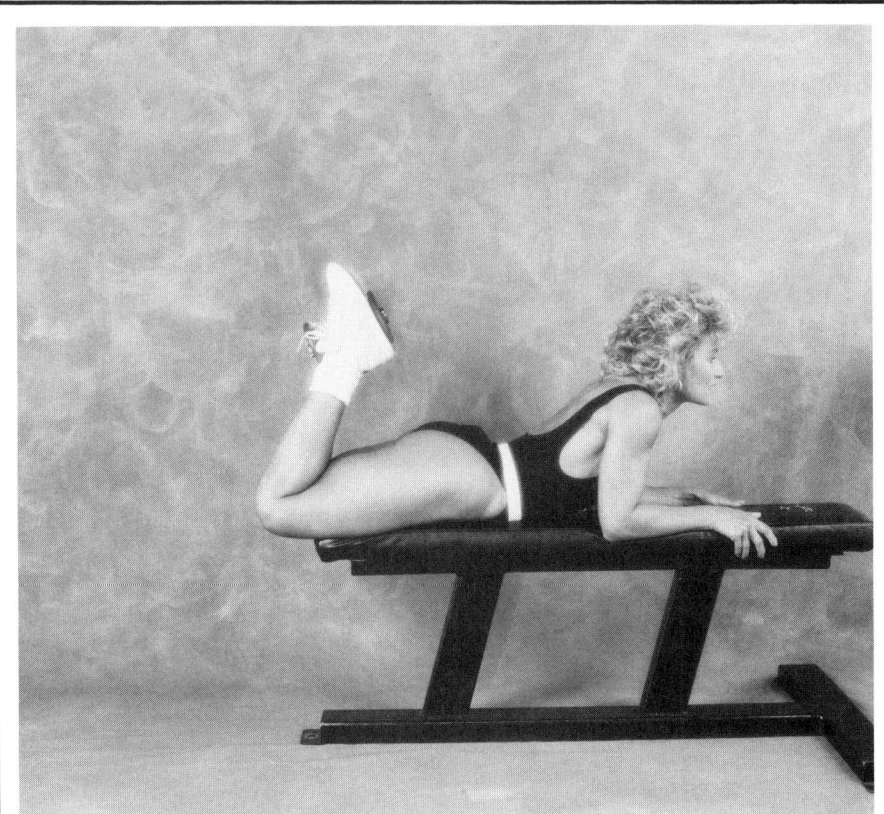

Finish

DAYS ONE, TWO, THREE, AND FOUR

ABDOMINAL ROUTINE

The abdominal area requires more work; fat tends to accumulate in this part of the female body. Because abdominal muscles respond better to high repetitions and light or no weights, you will be doing high reps and using little or no weight in these exercises.

You may start with ten repetitions for each set and work your way up to twenty-five repetitions, adding one rep each time you work out until you achieve the full twenty-five. If you are ambitious, you may work your way up to fifty repetitions. Even champion bodybuilders work their abdominal areas in this manner.

Straight Board Sit-ups— Abdominal Exercise #1

Follow the instructions on page 138.

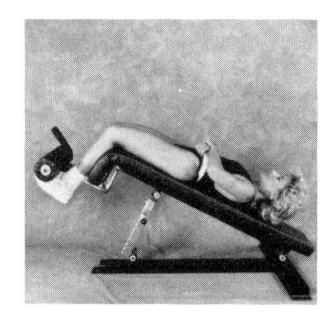

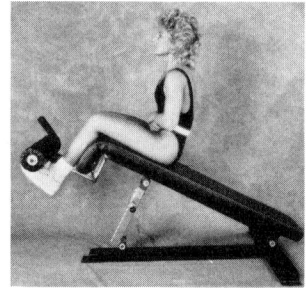

THE HOME WORKOUT **183**

Crunch— Abdominal Exercise #2

Follow the instructions on page 140.

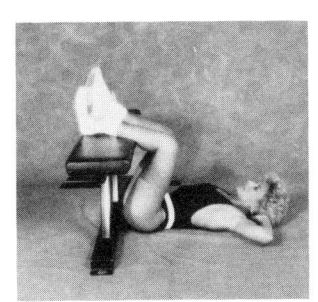

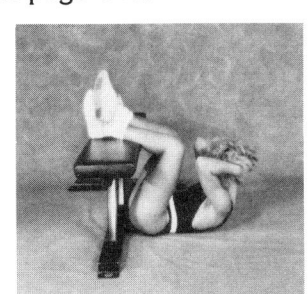

Bench Leg Raise with and without a Weight— Abdominal Exercise #3

Follow the instructions on page 142.

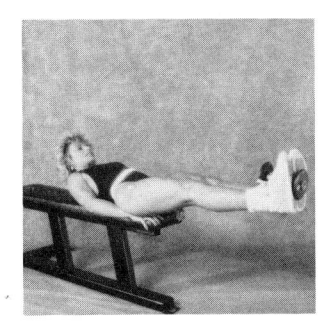

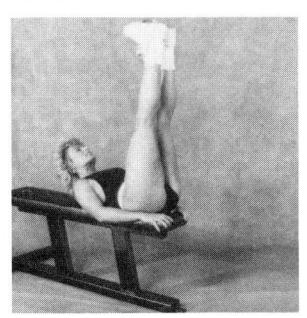

Leg-in with and without a Weight— Abdominal Exercise #4

Follow the instructions on page 144.

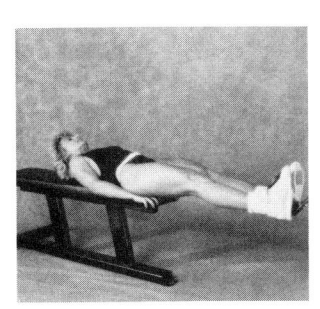

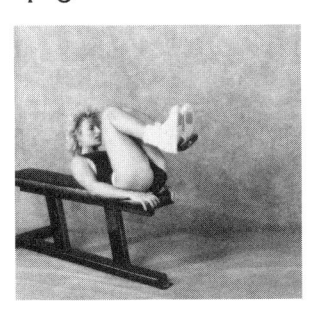

BUTTOCKS ROUTINE

The buttocks routine requires a special workout. Do not pyramid. Higher repetitions are required because fat tends to accumulate around that area. The basic formula for the buttocks is three sets of twenty-five repetitions for each exercise. If you wish to speed up your progress, you may do four sets of any or all of the exercises. (For more on "bombing," see Chapter 10.)

Start out with a light enough weight so that you can do fifteen repetitions of the exercise without too much difficulty. Add five repetitions a week until you can do each set with twenty-five repetitions.

After a month or two you may find that the weight is no longer a challenge. Change to the next higher weight. If you were using two pounds for your scissors exercise, for example, move up to five pounds. You may need to buy heavier ankle weights.

Remember, when doing buttocks exercises the heaviness of the weight is not as crucial as strict performance of the exercise and intense flexing of the buttocks muscle throughout the exercise.

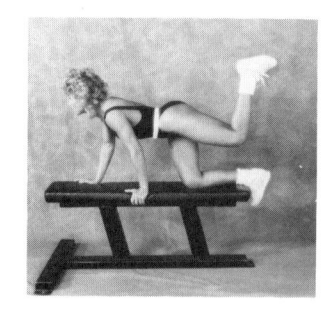

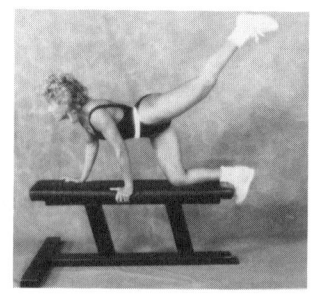

Feather Kick-up—Buttocks Exercise #1

Follow the instructions on page 146.

THE HOME WORKOUT

**Scissors—
Buttocks
Exercise #2**

Follow the instructions on page 148.

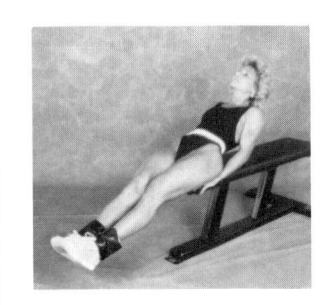

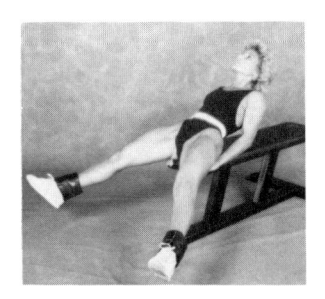

**Back Leg Kick—
Buttocks
Exercise #3**

Follow the instructions on page 150.

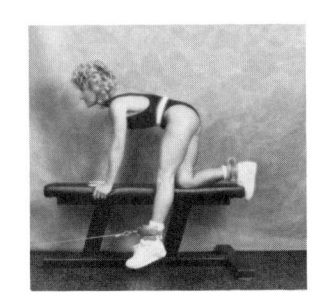

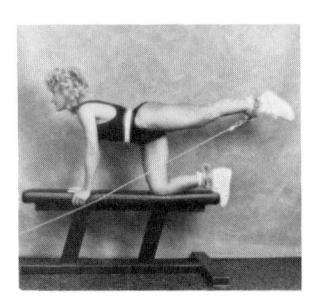

**Barbell Tuck—
Buttocks
Exercise #4**

Follow the instructions on page 152.

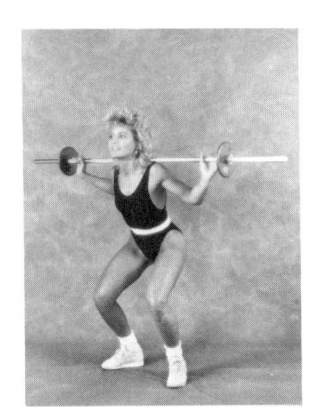

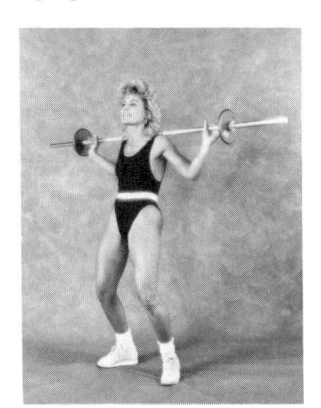

Photo by Bill Reynolds

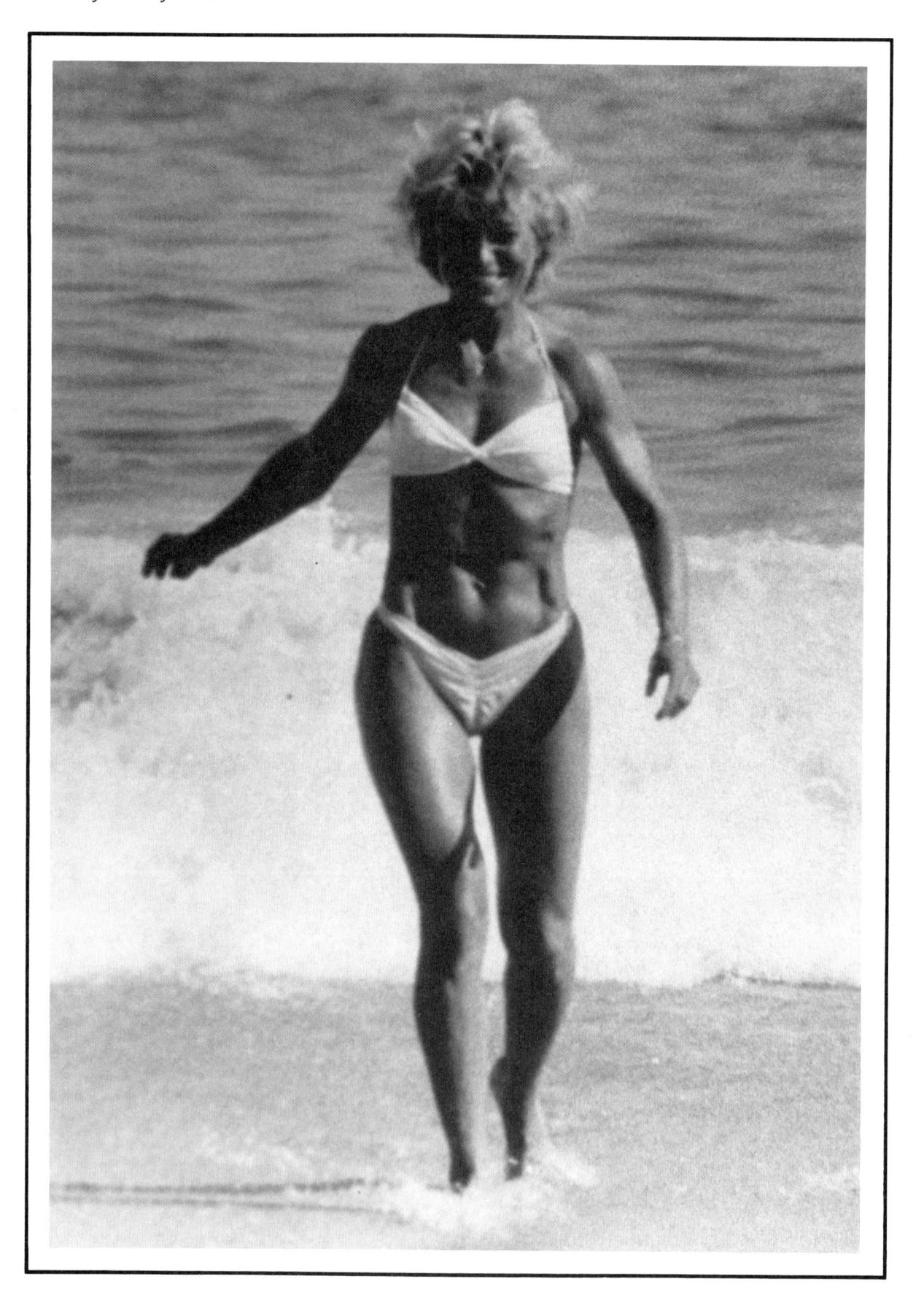

CHAPTER 9

DIET

The word *diet* has a bad reputation. It is associated with self-deprivation—hunger pangs, visions of forbidden foods, and continual guilt.

A new concept of dieting goes with this program. The emphasis is on foods that are delicious, nutritious, and satisfying. According to *Webster's Third International Dictionary*, your diet is simply your "usual food and drink." What will happen now is that your "usual" food and drink will change to "better than usual" food and drink—food and drink that is high in energy-producing potential and low in fat- and water-producing potential.

So yes, you will be on a diet. But this will not be a two-week plan or a five-day crash program. It will be a lifetime way of eating, an approach to nutrition that will become natural and "usual" for you. You will eat fresh fruits and vegetables, lean white-meat chicken and turkey, various fishes, and even pasta (with low-fat tomato sauce). Soon energy-sapping food toxins such as processed sugars (in every form—cookies, cakes, doughnuts, pie) and fat-loaded edibles (fried food, red meat, and ice cream) will cause your stomach to rebel. You will in fact develop a sort of Geiger counter for detection of food enemies and avoiding them will be easy. Your stomach will tell you when you make a mistake, and whenever you see an undesirable food item again, a negative sensation will cause you to say "no" to that food.

In time your system will become sensitive to high-sodium foods such as frankfurters, smoked fish, monosodium glutamate–loaded foods (Chinese foods are often heavily laced with MSG), and most canned items. Your taste buds will tell you to reject such foods, and you will learn to ask for food prepared without monosodium glutamate (Chinese restaurants will usually honor the request) and to eat fresh or frozen foods instead of canned foods.

NEW ADDICTIONS

We are all creatures of habit. When a habit is so ingrained that we refuse even to think in terms of giving it up, that can be seen as a form of addiction. If you are in the habit of eating a certain way, your body will at first fight a change. You will crave the missing foods and think that you must have them to survive. However, after the initial weaning period (about two months), you will come to enjoy the refreshing change in your diet. Soon you will become addicted to eating correctly—that is, relying on the foods that your body needs to function at optimum capacity. The bonus in this is that when you do become addicted to eating the foods your body really needs, your body will become even less willing to give up that diet. It will be very difficult for you to return to being a "junk food junkie," if that's what you were, even to take into your body a food poison such as a previously favored piece of layer cake. Your body will react angrily and may even give you a feeling of nausea.

For this very reason, I allow you to eat any forbidden foods you wish, once in a while. Your mind may tell you to have that thick shake or that greasy hamburger. Go ahead. Your body will cooperate to make sure it doesn't happen very often.

It is even a good idea to eat nonnutritious foods once in a while, just to give your body the opportunity to remind you that such foods are not what you really want. I eat a candy bar or an ice cream cone every so often, and once in a rare while I'll even have a thick, juicy steak. But these digressions from good eating are the exception rather than the rule, and that makes all the difference to your body.

HOW WE LOSE AND GAIN WEIGHT

Food energy is measured in calories. A calorie is the amount of chemical energy released when food is metabolized. Foods that contain lots of calories also contain lots of energy value. The problem arises when you do not use up all the energy potential being supplied by the calories. Your body stores the excess calories in the form of unwanted fat.

Out of the three main foods components, fat is the highest in calories. Whereas protein and carbohydrates yield 4 calories per gram, fat yields 9 calories per gram. It is easy to see that one will want to avoid fat in the diet if the goal is to lose body fat. In order to lose one pound of body fat, you must reduce your caloric intake by 3500 calories. Weight gain is achieved the same way, but in the reverse: You increase your caloric intake by 3500 calories.

The most intelligent way to lose weight is gradually, about one to two pounds a week. If you try to lose much faster than that, you will probably lose lean tissue. It is impossible for the body to give up more than about two to two and a half pounds of fat a week. Crash dieters may see a scale loss of as much as five or ten pounds in a week, but they don't realize that what they have lost is a lot of water, some fat, and some lean tissue (muscle). People who crash diet eventually become fatter than they were before the diet because of the loss of lean tissue. When they break the diet and the binge effect sets it, muscle is not put back on their frames, fat is. Muscle can only be developed by working out and eating the proper foods.

Muscle and Fat

Muscle weighs more than fat. Women who are very fat may not weigh as much as women who are not fat. Does that sound like a contradiction? It isn't. The scale, you see, is an instrument that measures only pounds. It is unable to distinguish between muscle and fat. Two women about five feet four inches can get on a scale, and both can weigh 140 pounds. One will look lean and shapely while the other will appear fat and out of shape. The lean and shapely woman may wear dresses two sizes smaller than those worn by her "fat" sister, despite their being the same height and weight.

Because of its dense consistency, muscle weighs more than fat. Your major concern will not be to lose weight but to lose fat. If you are very overweight now, chances are your scale weight will eventually go down, too, as you lose excess fat, but this should not concern you. Your main goal is to have a tight, lean, shapely body. What you see in the mirror will be your guide, not what you read on the scale.

Ideal Amount of Body Fat

A woman's body tends to produce more fat than a man's body because of the production of the female hormone estrogen. However, after age forty, estrogen production in women decreases, and with it the fat-holding tendency. This, of course, is in your favor. The ideal amount of body fat for you is about 20 percent or lower. Many women who are not overweight and look beautiful in a size seven dress are holding up to 35 percent fat on their bodies. In the nude the excess fat can be seen in the form of cellulite (bunched up fat) and feels soft, limp, and spongy to the touch. I have a friend who weighs 100 pounds and wears a size three dress, but she looks fat in a bikini. I am willing to bet that she is holding at least 35 percent of her weight as body fat on her petite frame. She will never get into shape unless she works out with weights to form muscle.

Perhaps you have heard that you cannot help but get fat once you pass a certain age. This myth was perpetuated for a good reason. Many people believe that they must "slow down" as they advance in years. They take this idea to the extreme and sit when they can stand, take the car when they can walk, take the elevator instead of the stairs, and do no physical exercise whatsoever. Remember how calories are spent—by exerting energy. Since such people are not spending their consumed calories, naturally fat accumulates on their bodies. Mentally they cooperate with the process of getting fat by saying to themselves, "This is what happens when you get old." They accept their "fate" and it becomes reality.

Since you are obviously of another ilk, you will reject such nonproductive thinking. Instead, you will mentally cooperate with the revitalization that takes place with the new stimulation of muscles that have been lying dormant for years. You will remind yourself that your body now tends *not* to store as much fat and that once you are lean, muscle burns more calories than fat, so you can actually consume more calories and not gain the fat you would add if you were fat.

WHAT FOOD IS MADE OF

There are three main sources of food energy: carbohydrates, proteins, and fats. In order to understand the principles of nutritious eating it is necessary to learn the basic facts about these food components.

Carbohydrates

Carbohydrates are the body's preferred energy sources. They are the main source of food for the brain and they help to metabolize protein and fat. A lack of carbohydrates in the diet causes listlessness and digestive problems, because without carbohydrates the fats in your body cannot be broken down properly in the liver.

There are three types of carbohydrates: processed, simple, and complex.

PROCESSED CARBOHYDRATES

These are the "bad guys" of the carbohydrate world. They include white flour and all processed sugars (notably sucrose, but also dextrose and others) such as can be found in:

cake	candy	puddings
cookies	presweetened	pastries
doughnuts	breakfast cereals	muffins
pie	syrup	
ice cream	jams and preserves	

In order to detect the presence of processed sugars, read food labels or look them up in *The Nutrition Almanac* (see bibliography).

Ingesting processed sugars gives you a quick lift because your blood sugar level rises immediately. This energy lift lasts about ten to twenty minutes, and then the blood sugar drops to a lower level than it was initially. This causes a sensation of weakness and fatigue. Sometimes you may experience this as a feeling of depression. Without realizing why, most people reach for another quick "fix" so they can achieve another boost. The trap here is evident. You can consume thousands of empty calories by continually adding quick sugars to the digestive system with the goal of getting energy—energy that doesn't last. Simple carbohydrates are a far better source of immediate energy, and complex carbohydrates are the best source of energy that will be gradually released during the day.

SIMPLE CARBOHYDRATES

Simple carbohydrates are found in all fruits. When ingested they go straight to the bloodstream and supply an immediate shot of energy without the price of a drop in the blood sugar level a few minutes later. Ideal simple carbohydrates can be found in fruits. Here are some choices:

cantaloupe	raspberry	grape	orange
cherry	blueberry	pear	honeydew melon
plum	peach	banana	tangerine
strawberry	pineapple	apple	nectarine

Some of the above-mentioned fruits are higher in calories than others. You will want to be aware of calories if you are on a weight-loss or weight-gain diet. Further details will be given later in this chapter.

COMPLEX CARBOHYDRATES

The best source of complex carbohydrates are vegetables, grains (especially whole grains), and pasta. They provide gradually released energy because of prolonged enzymatic action as they are broken down into simple sugars. Complex carbohydrates are more valuable than simple carbohydrates because they provide a natural continual energy supply for your workout and for your daily activities.

Excessive intake of carbohydrates (complex or simple) causes fat storage. After the conversion of simple and complex carbohydrates into glucose for use by the brain, nervous system, and muscles, the body stores a reserve in the muscles and liver as glycogen. If there is a surplus of glucose after that, it is stored in the body as fat. Eating too many calories, even in the form of good carbohydrates, leads to fat gain.

When you reduce your caloric intake, the body searches for fuel for energy. It focuses on excess fat and reconverts it into glucose, then uses it as energy. It is clear then that "losing weight," that is to say "fat," is really quite scientific. Reduce your caloric intake so that your body will be forced to draw on excess fat and burn it for essential energy.

Ideal complex carbohydrates can be found in the following foods:

peas	cauliflower	rice (white or brown)
carrots	spinach	pasta (whole wheat or high-protein)
green beans	potatoes	
squash	tomatoes	whole grain bread
	lettuce	

Protein

Muscles are composed mainly of protein, which is the main building material of the body. Hair, nails, skin, blood, and internal organs are all comprised of protein. The hormones that prompt sexual development are formed with the help of protein. Protein also affects growth, metabolism, and water balance in the body.

COMPLETE AND INCOMPLETE PROTEIN

Protein is made up of twenty-two elements called "amino acids." The human body can produce fourteen of these amino acids without the aid of an outside source, but the other eight must be obtained from certain foods. Foods that have all the needed amino acids are called "complete proteins," and those containing some but not all of the eight essential amino acids are called "incomplete proteins." Most of the complete protein comes from animal sources—poultry, red meat, fish, milk and milk products, and eggs. Although there are ways of combining two incomplete protein foods so as to make up a complete protein food, I do not recommend such combinations to fulfill your protein intake. Fortunately, in our country there are plenty of available complete protein sources. In countries lacking in complete protein sources people have traditionally made up a complete combination using rice and beans with corn and milk. There are other combinations as well. Vegetarians find it necessary to use such combinations to make up the complete protein requirement of a good diet. The most common sources of incomplete protein are corn, rice, beans, vegetables, nuts, seeds, and fruits.

You may be surprised to learn that even vegetables and fruits contain protein, but most contain such a minimal amount that it would be impossible to glean the needed supply from them.

Excessive protein intake at the expense of carbohydrates causes a phenomenon known as the "phosphorus jitters," a condition that makes one nervous and irritable. The high phosphorus content of protein, combined with its low calcium content, throws off the body's natural calcium-phosphorus balance to cause the phosphorus jitters. This condition is often experienced by those who foolishly try to lose weight quickly by following high protein–low carbohydrate fad diets. Protein intake must be balanced with the proper amount of carbohydrates and fat in the diet.

Fat

Most women think of fat as a food enemy, and for the most part it is. Yet it is also needed in our diet. Fat helps vitamins A, E, K, and D to be absorbed by the body, and it is responsible for the absorption of calcium into the body. If your diet lacked fat, your bones and teeth would suffer because calcium would not be properly absorbed into your body. In addition, fat serves as a cushion for internal organs such as the heart and lungs, preventing them from being injured with movement. Although too much fat under the skin is undesirable, a small amount is necessary to keep your body from losing heat too quickly. You may have noticed that extremely thin people tend to become cold and shiver more quickly than people with more fat on their bodies.

Of course, excessive intake of fat in any form can only result in the storage of unwanted fat. Yes, you are what you eat. Eat foods high in fat and you will inevitably become fat (or fatter). Eat foods that are lean and relatively fat free and you will inevitably become lean, with no more than a necessary minimum of fat on your body.

CHOLESTEROL

Cholesterol is a form of fat that is found in hard or solid form. It is present in red meats, cheese, and butter. Cholesterol is present in saturated fats (fats that appear in solid form) but not in unsaturated fats (those that appear in liquid form, such as vegetable oils and the like).

There is no need to concern yourself with cholesterol if you are planning to follow the good eating habits prescribed in this training program. Your cholesterol intake will automatically be limited to well below the unhealthy amount. You need never think about cholesterol again.

COMPOSITION OF THE IDEAL DIET

A balanced diet should consist of:

Carbohydrates	67%
Protein	18%
Fat	15%

A woman weighing 120 pounds and eating a balanced maintenance diet of 2000 calories would consume:

        Carbohydrates   1340 calories
        Protein   360 calories
        Fat   300 calories

The proportions have been carefully calculated to provide maximum muscle development, minimum fat accumulation, and maximum energy supply.

Most people consume well above the suggested amount of fat because they are unaware of the fat content of many foods. For example, one thick shake and an order of french fries will immediately place you over your fat limit for the day. There is enough fat found in "lean" foods such as white-meat chicken, an egg, or even an apple to supply your fat requirement for the day. (An average apple has 9 calories of fat; six ounces of broiled white-meat chicken has 68 calories of fat. Of course there are carbohydrate and protein calories in addition to the fat calories.) Getting enough fat in your diet will never be a problem, even when you eliminate all of the fat offenders.

The American diet also generally includes a much higher protein percentage than I recommend. The consumption of too much protein at the expense of carbohydrates results in poor digestion, since it is impossible to use more than twenty to thirty grams of protein at any one meal (80 to 120 calories of pure protein). The excess protein is eventually stored as fat. However, since you are working to build muscles, which are largely composed of protein, I recommend a slightly higher amount of protein in the diet than does Dr. Robert Haas.[1]

Because you get your fuel for energy from carbohydrates and the intake of certain carbohydrates can be timed to release energy steadily through the course of the day, I recommend a diet high in carbohydrates. But it should contain an absolute minimum of processed carbohydrates. You will have no trouble finding the right carbohydrates to fill your daily needs.

Sodium

Sodium is a necessary mineral. It regulates a healthy balance of fluids in the body and it prevents deposits of other minerals from building up in the bloodstream. In addition, sodium assists in balancing blood chemistry and aids the digestive processes and body purification of carbon dioxide. Those who lack sodium (virtually no one in the modern world) eventually experience difficulty with muscle contraction and expansion and proper nerve stimulation.

Almost every food contains sodium, and many foods contain too much for optimum health. The recommended amount of sodium intake is about 1200 to 1600 milligrams daily. Most people consume double or triple that amount, and such an overabundance of sodium causes the body to retain water. Sodium holds up to fifty times its own weight in water, so you can see that one would become quite bloated as a result of consuming high sodium foods such as a cup of regular cottage cheese (900 mg. sodium) or a six-ounce glass of tomato juice (500 mg. sodium). An individual consuming any high sodium foods at all will surely exceed the recommended daily amount of sodium, because anything one eats contains some sodium. For example, consider the following foods:

1 cup raw spinach	49 milligrams sodium
½ cantaloupe	24 milligrams sodium
6 ounces flounder	602 milligrams sodium
8 ounces chicken breast	140 milligrams sodium
1 cup raw lettuce	4 milligrams sodium

Although the above foods are highly recommended for our diet plan, even they contain sodium. You must learn to save your sodium "allowance" for such foods and not waste it on foods such as the following "sodium offenders":

Medium-sized pickle	930 milligrams sodium
Medium portion of chow-mein	1675 milligrams sodium
Burger King cheeseburger	563 milligrams sodium
Frankfurter	841 milligrams sodium
1 cup canned soup (average)	1000 milligrams sodium
1 cup canned vegetables (average)	400 milligrams sodium

Now that you know about sodium, you will want to avoid table salt altogether. One teaspoon of it contains 2000 milligrams of sodium. Never use it. Don't even put it into food when cooking. There are many tasty spices that can help you get out of the bad habit of excess sodium intake. Try spices such as:

dry mustard	sage	mace	nutmeg
marjoram	tarragon	fennel	mint
oregano	curry powder	rosemary	bay leaves
thyme	garlic powder	dill	sesame seed
ginger	onion powder	paprika	

You may also use vinegars of various flavors, as well as lemon juice and white and red cooking wines to give food an exciting flavor. See the bibliography for a book with low-salt, low-fat recipes (*Supercut* by Bill Reynolds and Joyce Vedral).

In general, watch out for all canned foods, fast foods, Chinese foods that contain MSG (and they all do unless you specifically request that it not be used), table salt, garlic or onion salt or any spiced salt, smoked foods, frozen dinners, frankfurters, knockwurst, salami, dried chipped beef, pizza, roast ham, potato chips, pretzels, and soy sauce. There are others. For an excellent little paperback on this, see the bibliography reference for *Shake the Salt Habit*.

Water

It is appropriate that the subject of water be discussed immediately after sodium, because water has been the victim of gross misunderstanding. Many people are under the misguided impression that if they drink a lot of water they will retain water. Actually, the opposite is true. Water flushes out your system. The more you drink, the more (in proportion to what you drink) you will eliminate. It is only when you eat a high-sodium diet that you retain water. And here is the surprise. The water you retain is not necessarily obtained from water you drink but rather from the water in the foods you eat. In other words, if your diet is high in sodium, even if you drink no water, your body will retain the water content in your food anyway. Even people on a high-sodium diet who drink lots of water do not retain more water than those who drink less. In fact, those who drink lots of water retain less, because pure water (bottled spring water, distilled water, or even tap water) flushes out the system.

Water is needed to cleanse your internal organs. It also functions to lubricate your skin and keeps your skin looking moist and young. A lack of water in the diet will inevitably show up in a dry, flaky skin tone. I saw a marked difference in my skin about three weeks after beginning to drink the right amount of water. People began to comment that I was looking younger. The comments, I believe, were more than a coincidence.

You should drink from six to eight eight-ounce glasses of water per day. This is plain water not included in coffee, soft drinks, or other beverages.

A side benefit of water is its ability to curb your appetite. The first thing you should do before you eat is drink a glass of water. I hate plain water so I squeeze in a lemon wedge so it goes down quite smoothly; I even enjoy it.

Forty-five to 55 percent of your body weight is comprised of water.[2] That amount of water is needed in the system because it is water that transports the nutrients throughout your body and helps to maintain your body temperature.

WEIGHT-LOSS DIET

In order to lose one pound of body fat, you must reduce your caloric intake by 3500 calories. If you reduce your caloric intake by 500 calories per day, you will lose one pound a week. In addition to that reduction, if you increase your energy expenditure by 500 calories per day, you will burn up an extra 3500 calories a week for the loss of another pound.

If you try to cut your calorie consumption too suddenly, your body will rebel and you will not be able to resist the urge to "binge." To avoid this I suggest that you figure out about how many calories a day you are presently consuming and then reduce that amount by 200 calories a day until you are eating between 1500 and 1800 calories. You should not plan to lose more than a pound to two pounds a week. The more slowly you lose weight, the more readily your body will accept the new body weight. Barbara Vale (see Before and After pictures, page 225) consumed 1800 calories a day.

Remember. You took a long time to gain the weight. At the time you were gaining, it may not have seemed that way because you were not in pain doing it. You were enjoying yourself. If you think back, you probably gained less than a pound a week on the average last year. (You didn't gain fifty-two pounds in a year, did you?) I am planning to keep you at your ideal body weight (within a few pounds) for life, so there's no need to rush weight loss and pay the price of swinging up and down the scale.

What to Eat

You must keep in mind the correct proportions of carbohydrate, protein, and fat intake. Remember, 67 percent of your intake will be in carbohydrates, 18 percent in protein, and 15 percent in fat. Since you will be allowed about 1500 calories, your caloric consumption should look like this:

Carbohydrates 1005 calories
Protein 270 calories
Fat 225 calories

CARBOHYDRATES

You will naturally want to choose from the lowest-calorie foods possible so that you can get the most for your calorie allowance. Here are some delicious low-calorie fruits and vegetables.

FRUITS *(Simple Carbohydrates)*

peach	cantaloupe	pineapple
grapefruit	raspberry	orange
strawberry	apple	plum

VEGETABLES

peas	carrot	squash
lettuce	tomato	turnip
pepper	spinach	green beans
potato	radish	cucumber
zucchini	asparagus	artichoke

You will also want to select some of your complex carbohydrates from pasta and grains. Here are some suggestions:

pasta (whole wheat, protein)	bran
rice (white or brown)	oatmeal
breads (whole wheat, protein)	puffed cereals (wheat and rice)

If you are in the mood to have something very sweet, indulge in higher calorie fruits such as cherries, bananas, and pears. A few additional calories in sweet fruits are far less damaging than a slew of nonnutritious calories in the candy bar you might eat instead.

PROTEIN

Select your protein requirement from the following low-calorie foods list. You may find others when you refer to *The Nutrition Almanac* or another, similar book.

white-meat chicken and turkey	sole
tuna in water, rinsed	flounder

FATS

You will have no problem finding sources for fats. Your main concern with fats will be determining how to limit them to the caloric allowance. Be sure to look up fat content of any foods you eat in your nutrition guide.

This diet, combined with your workout program, will net you an approximate one- to two-pound weight loss per week. In the beginning you may lose more weight, but much of that will be water loss because of your new low-sodium diet. This is good, but sustained gradual fat loss is what will get you to your goal of a firm, shapely lifetime body.

Accelerating Weight Loss

There are some special techniques which will encourage expeditious weight loss: additional aerobics, more frequent but reduced-quantity meals, timely low-calorie snacks, use of vinegar and lemon juice, "negative" and "positive" visualization, and self-induced metabolism speed-up.

ADDITIONAL AEROBICS

Weight loss can be accelerated by adding up to ten minutes to the three weekly aerobic sessions. This can, of course, be accomplished gradually. Many women become so excited about the progress they are making that they add an extra aerobic session or even two to their weekly routine. While this is unnecessary, it does get them to their weight-loss goal more quickly. Here are some caloric equivalents for aerobic workouts.

Aerobic dancing	600 calories per hour
Swimming	600 calories per hour
Skiing	600 calories per hour
Running	800 calories per hour
Jumping rope	800 calories per hour
Riding stationary bicycle	700 calories per hour
Playing racquetball	450 calories per hour
Walking briskly	400 calories per hour

If you choose to throw in an extra workout day, you will burn about 400 additional calories per half hour. All of the above calculations are estimates and are based upon the assumption that you move vigorously. If you move very slowly, deduct 200 calories per hour from each of the exercises listed.

MORE FREQUENT BUT REDUCED-QUANTITY MEALS

Increasing the number of times you eat can help shift your metabolism "into gear" more often, with the result that you burn more calories. For example, instead of eating all of your daily caloric allowance in three meals, split it up into five meals. What happens is somewhat like what happens with fuel in a car engine. If you start the motor up five times, more fuel is burned than if you started the motor up only three times. People who are trying desperately to lose weight often punish themselves into having only one meal a day, and that in the evening. They are doing the worst possible thing for their weight-loss program.

Eating just once a day not only causes the inefficient burning of food energy, it causes overeating. The body is fooled into believing that it is starving and demands more food, sometimes insisting on "bad" foods. Also, the temptation to eat all evening long will be almost irresistible. Finally, eating heavily just before bedtime is never a good idea because the food is not metabolized as it would be during periods of activity. When one sleeps, one's metabolism usually slows down, too.

SNACKS

In addition to five well-spaced light meals, there are some calorie-free snacks available for the dieter. Fresh lettuce dressed with vinegar, herbal tea, or some carrot sticks will do no harm if you are feeling the need to eat something extra. Soda water or diet drinks sweetened with NutraSweet are also fair game.

VINEGAR AND LEMON JUICE

Vinegar and lemon juice are catalysts for fat burning. Try to develop a taste for them. Vinegars come in all sorts of flavors today (red wine, tarragon, garlic, apple cider, etc.). Pour vinegar onto anything: lettuce, broiling fish, low-sodium cottage cheese, etc. You'll be amazed how delicious foods can taste with this new flavoring.

Do the same with lemon juice. Add a wedge of squeezed lemon to every glass of water you drink.

NEGATIVE AND POSITIVE VISUALIZATION

Dr. Donald Wilson describes a very effective method of helping yourself to love nutritious foods and to reject food enemies.[3] He tells you to sit in front of a dining room table and imagine the table filled with fattening foods such as cakes, ice cream, fried foods, etc. He then tells you to visualize on the same table nutritious foods such as fresh vegetables, lean meats, and delicious fruits. Next he directs you to see yourself getting a strong urge to eat only the foods that are good for you. See yourself starting to eat some of the foods that are good for you and feel the delicious taste of them in your mouth. Then picture yourself pushing away the fattening foods in disgust. Make up your own list of food "demons" and do this exercise regularly.

Dr. Paul E. Wood describes his experience with a client using visualization. The story speaks for itself.*

> Mrs. Kay was a typical overweight middle-aged housewife who had tried every diet on the market....

---

*From *How to Get Yourself to Do What You Want to Do* by Paul E. Wood. Copyright © 1981 by Paul E. Wood. Reprinted by permission of the publisher, Prentice-Hall, Inc., Englewood Cliffs, New Jersey 07632. The italics are mine.

> I instructed Mrs. Kay that she was to eat anything she wanted and that she did not have to do any exercise. All she had to do was deeply relax and visually imagine herself actually the size and shape she desired....Mrs. Kay was determined to be successful this time and practiced the relaxation and imagery up to ten times a day in the first week. She reported a two-pound weight loss in the first week and felt disappointed....She was further instructed in the technique of seeing herself standing in front of a "magic mirror" which showed her in vivid detail exactly the size, shape, and proportion she desired....
>
> Mrs. Kay slowly and progressively began losing weight, and her body realigned itself to a new figure. Unconsciously and effortlessly, Mrs. Kay *found herself avoiding fattening foods. At the same time, she developed an interest in active exercises,* beginning with walking and moving up to jogging and bike riding, eventually enrolling in a dance exercise class....
>
> Ultimately Mrs. Kay lost eighty-five pounds, leveling off at a good weight for her body build.

Notice that Mrs. Kay, although told that she did not have to diet or exercise, nevertheless began dieting and exercising. Her eating habits changed and she began naturally to take an interest in exercising. Once the mind is given instructions to achieve a certain goal, it works like a guided missile with a program to follow and zigzags its way toward its goal, doing whatever is necessary to get there.

SPEEDING UP YOUR METABOLISM

Many researchers today are coming to realize that the mind controls the body to a much greater extent than ever imagined. You can mentally speed up your metabolism by imagining an "on" switch that causes your body to double its food burning capacity. You can do this to your metabolism any time, day or night. You can lie in your bed at night and turn your metabolism "on." Picture a machine inside your stomach turning on and beginning to burn fat all night long. It works. Try it. You may even feel your skin tingling as you sleep.

THE WEIGHT-GAIN DIET

In order to gain a pound of weight, it is necessary to increase your caloric intake by 3500 calories. In order to ensure that the increased caloric intake results in muscle gain rather than fat gain, you must be sure to consume the additional calories in simple and complex carbohydrates and protein and eat a minimum of additional fat. It is also necessary to work out with weights as prescribed in this program.

The healthiest way to increase your caloric intake is to raise your consumption of calories by 150 to 200 a day until you have reached an additional caloric consumption of 500 a day or 3500 a week.

What to Eat

Keeping in mind the correct proportions of carbohydrate, protein, and fat intake (67 percent, 18 percent, and 15 percent) select from the following foods:

CARBOHYDRATES

All fresh fruits, *particularly*

Cherries
Bananas
Dates
Watermelon
Pears
Plantain
Avocado

All fresh vegetables, *particularly*

Corn
Beets
Sweet potato

Others

Bran and corn muffins
Bagels
Any grain product on the weight-loss list

PROTEIN

Meat

Lean beef
Liver
Dark-meat turkey and chicken

Fish

Bluefish
Salmon
Mackerel

When selecting the additional 500 calories for your daily increased consumption you should choose most of them from the complex carbohydrate group. These are the most economical calories for your body because such calories are gradually released for muscle fuel.

The additional protein intake (within the 18 percent caloric allowance) will immediately be invested in building shapely muscle so that your body will appear curvaceous rather than boney and saggy.

MAINTENANCE LIFE-STYLE DIET

Once you reach your ideal weight, you may follow these guidelines for lifetime eating. Keep your food choices within the general guidelines.

Carbohydrates	67%
Protein	18%
Fat	15%

Assuming you are following the workout plan given in this book and have an average metabolism, your daily calorie allowance is as follows (look at the chart for your ideal maintenance level):

Maintenance Weight	**Calories Allowed**
100 pounds	1700
110 pounds	1825
120 pounds	1950
130 pounds	2050
140 pounds	2200
150 pounds	2300

If you begin overeating, you can expect to gain weight. If you want to know how much you will weigh after a year of overeating on the level of, say, 2050 calories, you can see by the above chart that you will weigh about 130 pounds in time. (This assumes an average metabolism.)

Some women can eat more than the above allowance and still maintain their ideal weight level. This is because they have a faster metabolism. I can eat about 2500 calories and maintain a body weight of about 120 pounds.

Another reason some women can eat more than others and still maintain their ideal weight level is physical activity. Without even realizing it, some people are naturally more active than others. For example, one person will sit whenever an opportunity arises, while another will stand; some will choose to walk, while others will take the car; and so on. In addition, some people engage in additional physical activities—tennis, golf, badminton, swimming, etc.—on a regular basis, while others do not.

In order to find your actual maintenance level you will have to experiment for a while. The above chart is merely a general guideline.

You may choose from any and all of the savory foods suggested for either the weight-loss or weight-gain diets, and feel free to eat any other nutritious food that appeal to you.

Even "forbidden" foods are occasionally permissible. Everyone likes to eat a forbidden food once in a while. That is fine as long as you make it the exception rather than the rule. A thick shake, a greasy hamburger, half of a pizza, two slices of apple pie, or gravy on buttery mashed potatoes now and then will not ruin you *if your basic diet is under control*. You can even eat anything you want guilt-free on occasions such as Thanksgiving, Christmas, or a special weekend now that you have a sense of good eating habits for daily life.

Freedom from Fear of Weight Gain

Now that you have a basic knowledge of how you gain and lose weight, you need never panic again when you gain a few pounds. Simply begin to follow the weight-loss diet. Some women allow themselves to put on as much as five to seven pounds in the winter and then begin dieting in early spring. If you wish to do this, there is no reason not to, now that you are in control of what happens to your body. Food is no longer a mystery, and you now understand the processes of weight gain and weight loss.

I generally allow myself to gain about seven pounds in the winter. I like to eat more in the winter, and it's worth the price of later dieting to me. I have learned from many years' experience that the excess weight will be eliminated from my body in a scientific, systematic fashion as soon as I adjust my eating habits. I can always do some extra aerobics on a regular basis to speed up the weight-loss process. I adjust my diet to lose a pound a week—no more—until I achieve my ideal weight.

The beauty of this approach to weight gain and weight loss is peace of mind. One need never again become desperate at evidence of weight gain. Instead, one simply makes an intelligent decision about when to cut back on calories just enough to lose one pound a week.

Mental Weight Setting

Give yourself an ideal weight and then set off an automatic mental alarm when you go more than a certain amount over that weight. My alarm goes off in the winter when I am more than seven pounds over ideal weight and in the summer when I am more than three pounds over ideal weight.

As soon as you exceed your three-to-seven-pound limit, begin following the weight-loss diet.

A Bonus for the Muscular Woman

It has been discovered that a muscular body metabolizes food more quickly than does a fat body, even at rest. In other words, a fat body is naturally sluggish and burns calories inefficiently. A muscular body is naturally dynamic and burns calories efficiently.

Once you achieve a low body fat level and you are at your ideal weight, you can look forward to burning more calories just sitting in a chair and reading than you used to when you were fat. For example, a fat person will burn about 60 calories an hour while reading, but a person with low body fat will burn about 80 calories an hour reading. A person with an in-between amount of body fat will burn about 72 calories an hour reading.

The bonus for those who work out and put on muscle while reducing body fat is an ability to eat more than before without gaining weight. No longer will you be one of those women who are close to the truth when they say, "All I have to do is look at food and I get fat." Your naturally heightened metabolism will allow you to eat a little more without having to work the extra calories off with the penance of additional exercising.

DIET CAUTIONS

Fad Diets

Any diet that promises quick weight loss (more than two pounds a week) is a fad diet. The inevitable end result of such diets is additional fat gain. Fad diets prescribe unbalanced eating, which causes a natural "binge" reaction. Trying to resist this urge is like trying to fight the tide. The survival instinct of the body, triggered by the diet regimen, will win out in the end and push you into binging before you can begin eating intelligently again. The binge usually takes as long as the diet itself plus a day or two.

Alcohol

Although a glass of wine with dinner can be refreshing, in general alcohol has little place in a healthy lifetime diet. You can have a drink or two with some friends on a rare occasion, but be sure to select a nonmixed drink (have it with club soda or water).

The calories you consume while imbibing alcohol are nonnutritious and fall under the category of processed carbohydrates. In addition, alcohol is a depressant, and if you drink enough you will let down your guard and eat foods that ordinarily you would shun.

Finally alcohol has a negative effect on your energy level. Chances are you will feel the difference the next day when you are running or working out in the gym if you had more than two drinks the night before. However, a bonus comes to you in this very area just because you *are* working out. You will find that your body tends to reject excessive drinking. It will "know better" than to overindulge, because it will "remember" what happened the last time you had "a few." You will find yourself tempering your drinking without even knowing why on a conscious level. I have discussed this subject with many women who follow this program, and they all agree that their alcohol consumption has been reduced to little or nothing, and some of them previously drank quite a bit (either at business lunches or on the weekends).

Eating before a Workout

"Something was wrong with me yesterday," said Dorothy, age forty-three. "I felt nauseous and I couldn't do my abdominal routine. I had to leave the gym." After a series of questions I discovered that she had eaten a heavy lunch one-half hour before she began working out.

Eating less than an hour and a half before a workout will certainly cause nausea. If you *must,* have a light snack up to a half hour before, but not more than a slice of toast or a piece of fruit. Save your eating for about *an hour after* your workout. (If you eat immediately after a workout, you will upset your stomach because your metabolism is occupied with restoring your body to homeostasis.)

The nausea caused by Dorothy's eating occurred because her metabolism was busy digesting food and was unavailable to pump the necessary blood supply to the muscles being exercised. In addition, Dorothy's stomach simply had too much food in it, so when she jarred it up and down in sit-up and crunch movements, it became queasy.

POINTS TO REMEMBER

★ A diet is not a punishment.

★ Your body will become addicted to nutritious foods.

★ Eat a balanced diet composed of 67 percent carbohydrates, 18 percent protein, and 15 percent fat.

★ Read food labels and purchase a nutrition almanac or guide.

★ Avoid "sodium enemies."

★ Avoid "fat enemies."

★ Avoid "sugar enemies."

★ Use spices, vinegar, and lemon juice.

★ Drink lots of water.

★ Limit alcohol intake.

★ Lose weight slowly, one to two pounds a week.

★ Visualize your body goal.

★ Remember weight loss is a scientific process. Never panic.

★ Set a mental weight-gain limit that triggers an alarm.

1. Dr. Robert Haas, *Eat to Win: The Sports Nutrition Bible* (New York: Rawson Associates, 1983), pp. 19–20. Dr. Haas recommends forty to eighty grams of protein a day (160 to 320 calories). The higher amount would apply to people weighing more and who legitimately consume more calories. His percentage of protein works out to be about 10 percent, as opposed to my recommendation of about 18 percent. Dr. Haas and I are in agreement regarding the necessity of high carbohydrate intake for energy supply.

2. Irene Beland, R.N., M.S., and Joyce Y. Passos, R.N., Ph.D., *Clinical Nursing: Pathophysiological and Psychosocial Approaches*, 4th Edition (New York: Macmillan, 1981), p. 397.

3. Dr. Donald Wilson, M.D., *Total Mind Power* (New York: Berkley Books, 1978), pp. 86–89.

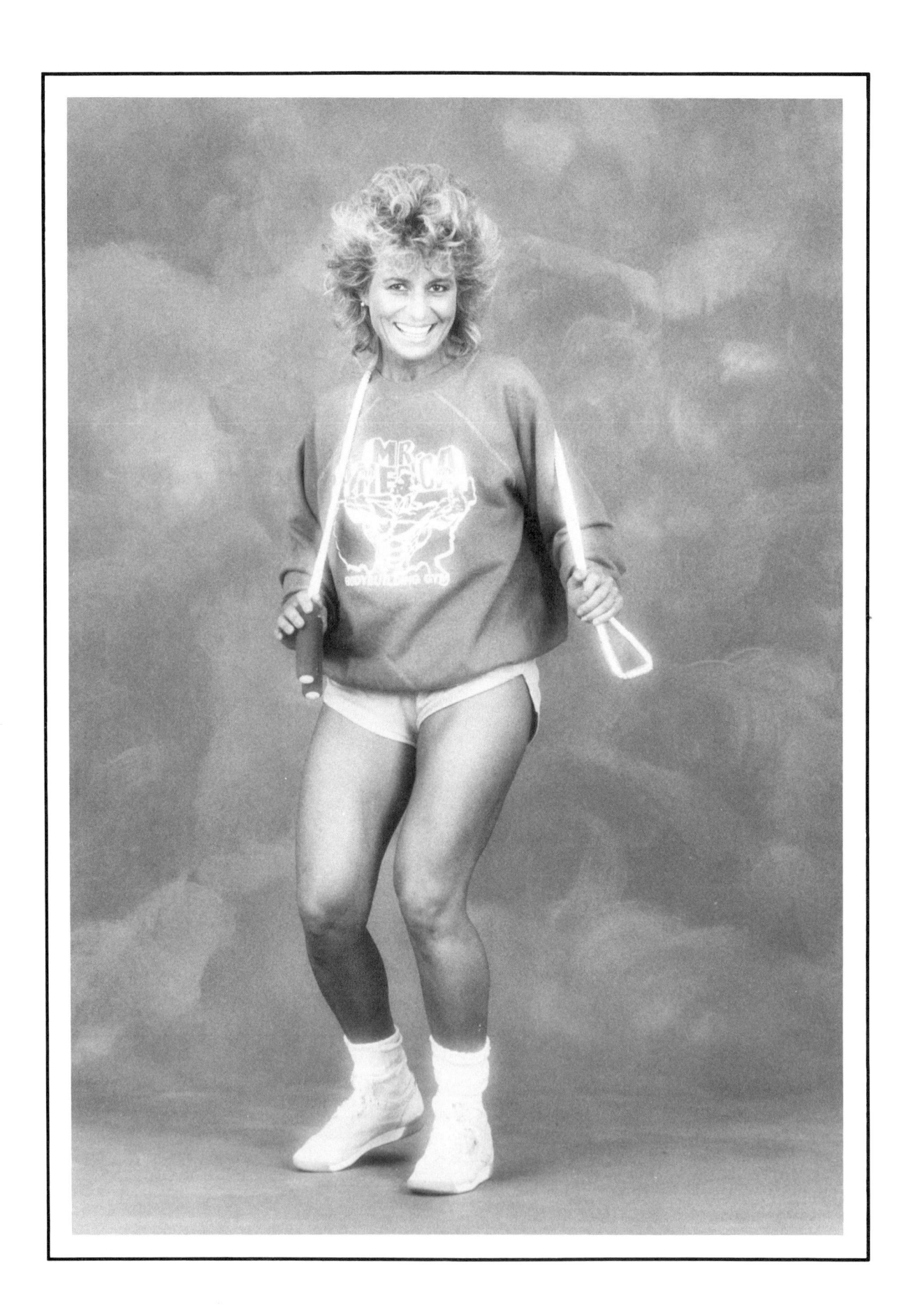

CHAPTER 10

BOMBING PROBLEM AREAS

You may be having a lot of trouble perfecting a certain area. If so, this chapter will tell you what additional methods to employ to correct that area.

Or you may be reading this chapter because you wish to concentrate on one body part, an area that you particularly wish to change. You don't want to follow the entire workout program. If this is the case, you will be happy to hear that, contrary to the myth that "it is impossible to spot reduce," you can indeed do just that.

The saying that you can't spot reduce is based on a truth—it is impossible to spot reduce by dieting. If you diet, fat is removed from all over your body, not just your abdominal area, for example. If, however, you work out with weights and concentrate exclusively on a particular area, muscle is formed there and some fat is worn away. You do indeed change that area. The only reason you would not see changes there would be that you are more than ten pounds overweight and the area is covered with so much fat that the muscles you are forming by working out are not visible. However, they would still be there, and when you lost weight so that the fat layer hiding them was reduced, the muscles in the spot you worked would show up.

Martha, a sixty-one-year-old retired telephone operator, has been following this workout program for only her triceps, and in four months she has seen remarkable results. She is about to add shoulders to her routine. It's my guess that she will soon be doing a full body workout.

Although I do not advise people to pick just one body part and work it, there is no reason not to do that if you merely want to see what happens when you work that one area. If you want to try this, turn to the pages in the gym or home workout that apply to the area you are interested in altering, do those exercises, and then follow the additional suggestions given in this chapter for that body part.

If you are already following the full body program given earlier in this book, follow the suggestions given here for additional progress on a troublesome body part. However, I recommend using bombing techniques only after about six months to a year, because until then you'll still be making remarkable progress with the regular routine. If you are impatient, you can start after three months. It certainly can't hurt you, even if it may not yet be necessary for ensuring progress.

MUSCLE PRIORITY TRAINING

If you have a troublesome body part, begin your training day with that body part. For example, if your problem area is your buttocks, instead of starting Training Day One with the chest exercises, start with the buttocks exercises. Instead of starting Training Day Two with the biceps exercises, begin again with buttocks exercises. By giving your troublesome area your first shot of energy, you will be training that area harder and more precisely than you would had you left it until later in your routine.

TRAINING TO FAILURE

The expression *training to failure* refers to the practice of working a body part to the point of exhaustion. There are three ways to do this. Each method forces the muscle to work as hard as possible causing a maximum amount of blood to be pumped into the body part.

Cheating

Perhaps the only time you will be allowed to cheat legitimately will be when you use this bodybuilding technique. The term *cheating* was coined by Joe Weider, trainer of champion bodybuilders, to describe a method of getting a few more repetitions from a set once the required number of repetitions have been completed. This is accomplished at the expense of strict form. For example, in the leg extension, cheating allows the individual to swing the weight up slightly rather than slowly raise it and to return to the start position quickly rather than slowly for those few extra repetitions. The purpose of this is to push the muscle beyond a former exertion limit.

If your problem area is your triceps and you wish to employ the method of cheating, do a few extra reps at the end of the last set of each triceps exercise. If your problem area is abdominals, do a few extra reps at the end of your final set of each abdominal exercise. If your problem area is buttocks, do a few extra reps for your final set of each buttocks area. In each case, follow strict form until you can't manage another rep that way, then allow yourself to cheat on form for the extra reps.

Forced Repetitions

Forced repetitions can be looked at as a form of cheating, only this time someone else is involved in the cheating—he or she helps you to get a few more reps at the end of a set by lending very slight assistance. For example, if you are doing triceps pushdowns, you ask someone to spot you for a few extra reps. That person slightly pushes the bar for you. You are still doing most of the work, but the slight assistance from the helper makes it possible for you to break through your previous exertion limit. This helps the muscle grow and respond. Use this method in the last set of each exercise for your troublesome area. Naturally, you will want to choose between cheating and forced reps.

Burns

Burns involve more actual cheating on strict form than either cheating or forced reps. A burn involves shortening the movement of the exercise to about one-half of the normal range and quickly repeating half movements until you feel a burning sensation in the muscle. The burning sensation comes from a buildup of lactic acid in the muscle tissue which the blood can't carry away as fast as it forms during constant movement.

When using this technique, first perform the required number of repetitions for your set in the strictest possible form. Only then begin doing burns. For example, if you are performing the triceps pushdown, after your last perfectly performed repetition, move the triceps bar up and down about half the normal distance as many times as possible until you feel a burning sensation in the muscle. Then stop. You may do burns for all three sets of each exercise.

How to Use Training-to-Failure Techniques

There are two ways to employ these techniques: Either do one of the above for your last set of each exercise or add an additional light set to your prescribed three sets and use the technique for that last additional light set. This new set will be the same as your first set. For example, if you are doing triceps pushdowns, and your first set is fifteen repetitions at twenty pounds, your second set ten repetitions at twenty-five pounds, and your third set six to eight repetitions at thirty pounds, do your fourth set for fifteen repetitions or more at twenty pounds, using either cheating, forced repping, or burning. You must choose just one of the three training-to-failure methods, as it is impossible to perform more than one per exercise. However, it is a good idea to vary the training-to-failure techniques from time to time, using one for a week and then switching to another.

ADDITIONAL SETS

Another way to attack troublesome areas is simply to add an additional set to the exercises for that area. For example, if your troublesome area is your chest, you add an additional set to each chest exercises, following the pyramid progression. For example:

Bench Press
1. 15 reps, 20 pounds
2. 12 reps, 30 pounds
3. 10 reps, 50 pounds
4. 6–8 reps, 60 pounds

Follow this pattern for all additional set plans.

Many women add the additional set to their entire workout (except biceps and triceps, more than twelve sets for those body parts is counterproductive—it wears away muscle). This would add about twenty minutes to your workout time, but it would also accelerate your progress and burn additional calories.

ADDITIONAL DAYS

Finally, you can go to the gym an extra day or two or work at home an extra day or two on the troublesome body part *only*. For example, if your regular training days are Monday, Tuesday, Thursday, and Friday, you can go to the gym or train at home on Saturday, Sunday, or Wednesday. Many women do the abdominal and buttocks routines two additional days. Most perform the routine at home rather than go to the gym an additional day. (See the home workout section for the appropriate exercise directions.)

COMMON TROUBLESOME AREAS

The most complained about area on women is the abdominal area. Running a close second is the buttocks-hip-thigh area,[1] and in third place is triceps. Chest (sagging breasts) ranks fourth. In order to "bomb" any of these areas, do the following:

1. Train the troublesome area first in your training day.
2. Use one of the training-to-failure methods on the troublesome body part.
3. Add an additional set to each exercise for your troublesome body part.
4. Train the troublesome body part one or two additional days.

---

1. The buttocks-hip-thigh area is grouped together because the exercises that work the buttocks also work the hips and thighs, and the exercises that challenge the hips and thighs also stress the buttocks. For example, a squat, which works the thigh muscle, also stresses the buttocks muscle; a feather kick-up, which works the buttocks muscle, also works the hip-thigh area; etc.

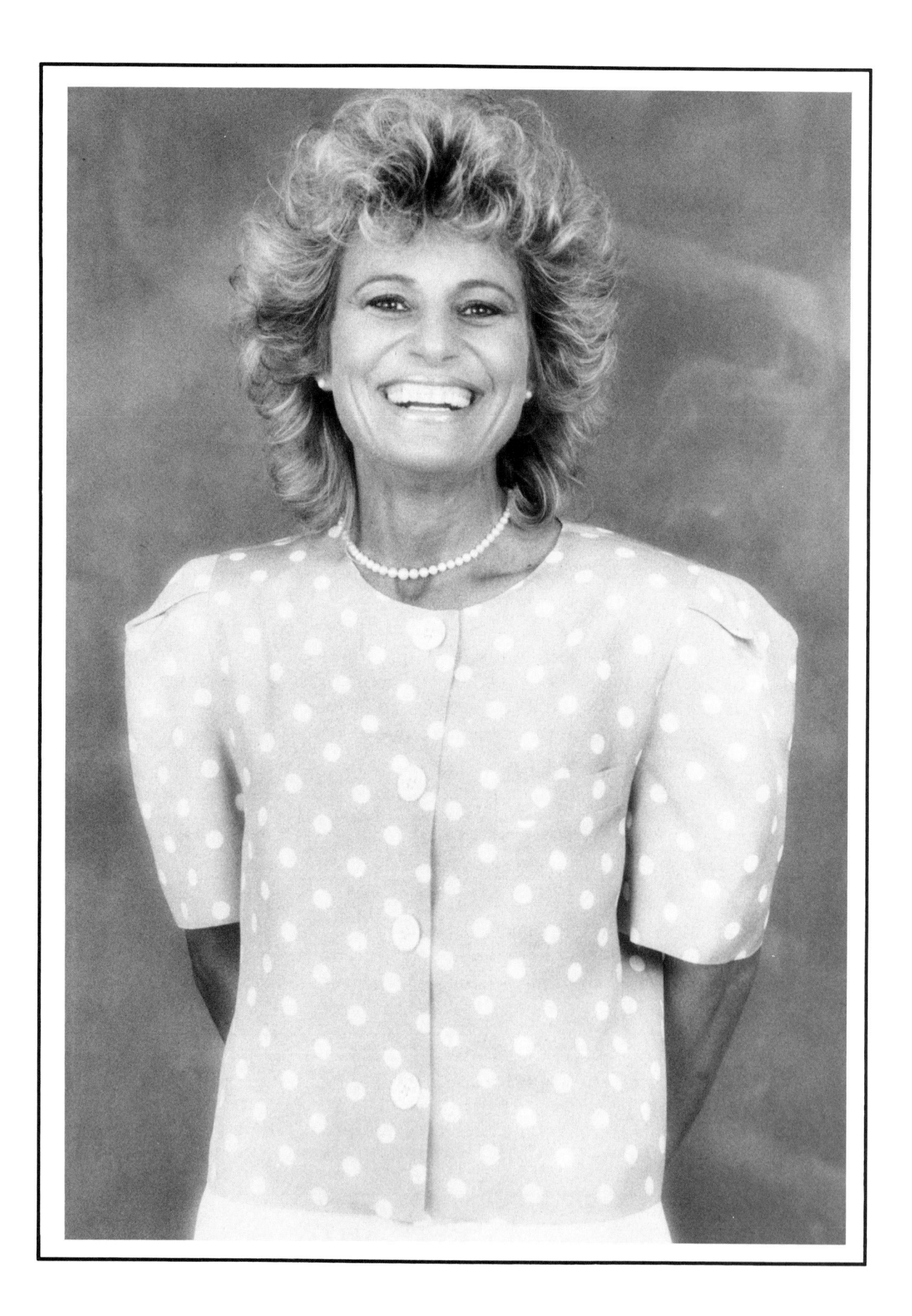

CHAPTER 11

BEFORE AND AFTER

You picked up this book because you are dissatisfied with your body. Perhaps you've told yourself, "There is no hope. It's too late. I'm too old." And yet you hope.

It is *not* too late. You are *not* too old. You *can* build yourself a more attractive, younger-looking body.

And here's the evidence to prove it.

Each of the four women profiled in this chapter thought there was no hope for her. Each tried various diets and sports and fitness programs, with little or no results. Fortunately, each persisted in the pursuit of her goal and finally discovered the program I've presented in this book for body transformation.

Look at the "before" picture in each case, and then compare that to the "after" picture. See the difference a scientific body-shaping program can make.

This program can make that kind of difference for you. Become an "after." It will take you less than a year.

TAKE A "BEFORE" PICTURE

Do yourself a favor and take a "before" picture. You may hesitate, thinking, "I can't bear to see my body in a permanent picture looking the way it does." Overcome this feeling and take the picture. Then paste it into the space provided for your "before" (see page 227). Just like the four women shown here, you will soon be an "after." Take the picture with a bikini if you dare, or at least a bathing suit or leotard.

Those women who refuse to take a "before" are invariably sorry later. They wish they had a record of how drastically their bodies have changed. Anne, a thirty-four-year-old lawyer, says, "Now that I'm in shape I wish I hadn't been so ashamed of my body before. I wouldn't let anyone photograph me in shorts, much less a bathing suit." Anne, like many other women, could not be included in this book because she couldn't supply a "before."

It's a good idea to take a picture of yourself every three months so you can see your quarterly progress—four steps to a year's goal, the perfect body.

ROBERTA ROBINSON, 43

Roberta weighed 117 pounds in the "before" picture. Although she was twenty-six then, when she started this program at the age of forty-two, she looked basically the same, only older, and she was the same weight, 117. In her "after" picture Roberta is forty-three and weighs 107 pounds. (You may be thinking that she looks a lot heavier than 117 in her "before" picture if she's only 10 pounds less in her "after" picture. But remember: Muscle weighs more than fat.)

The mother of three children ranging in age from six to twenty-three, she was a housewife when she started this program. Now she is enrolled in a school where she is training to become a qualified fitness instructor.

"I tried every diet you can name, and I did a lot of dancing—especially Middle Eastern dancing—but nothing really changed the shape or quality of my body. I had lots of cellulite and a pot belly, plus a rear end that was diving to the pavement."

Roberta admits that it wasn't easy to get started. But once she passed the first few weeks, "it actually got easier. Things became automatic.

"What really kept me going was the results I began to see after about a month. I saw my arms and chest developing. Then I realized that other parts would develop, too. I got hooked. Now if I miss a workout I feel terrible. I miss the feeling you get, and the results as well."

BEFORE AND AFTER

Before (117 pounds)

After one year
(107 pounds)

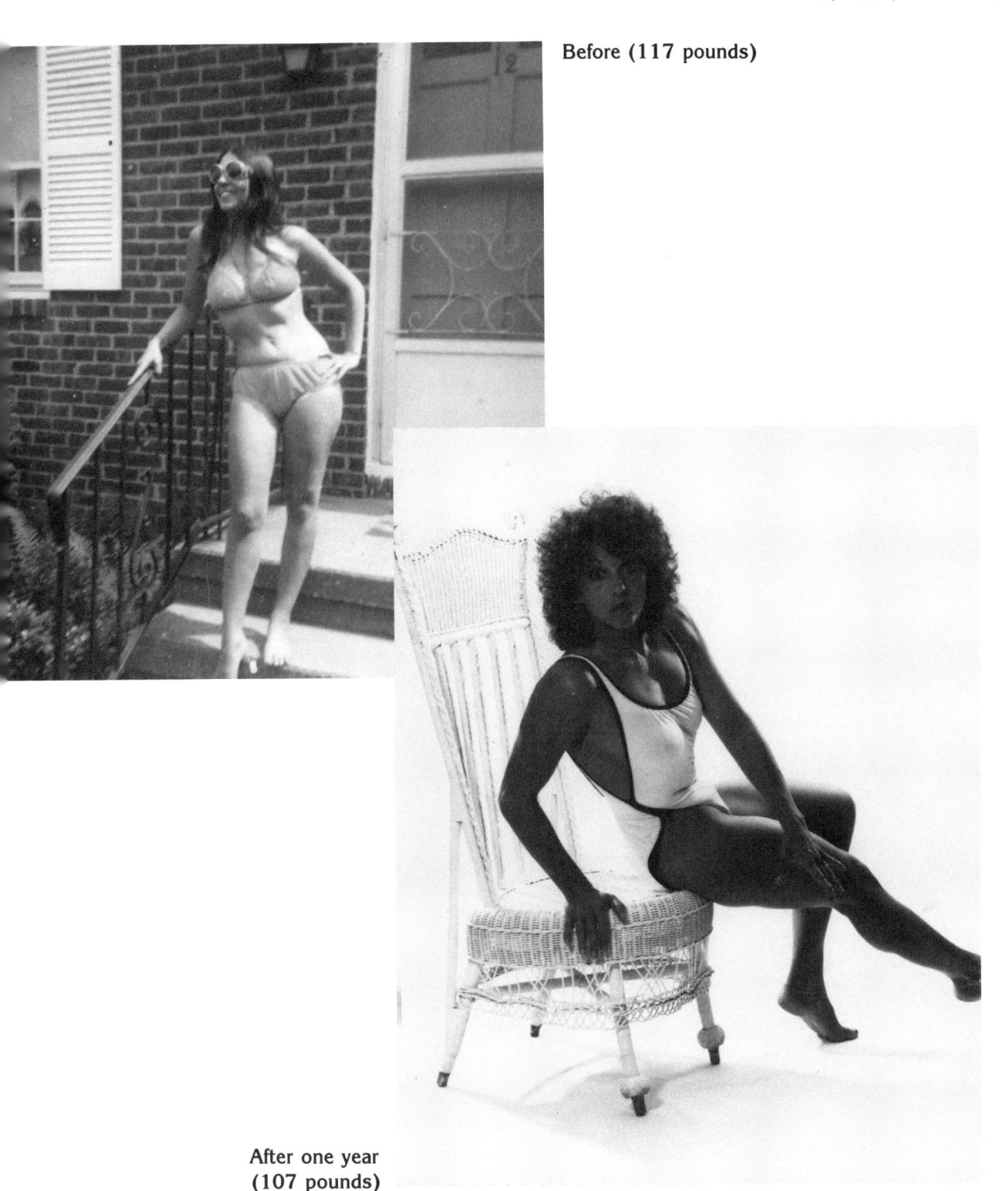

Bodybuilding has given Roberta more than just a new body. "I am so excited about goals now. I see that with deliberation and time I can achieve just about anything. Also, working out provides me with a release from stress. When I go to the gym I leave my worries behind. What I do here is not connected to anything or anyone else. It's totally my time."

TERRY PERINE, 44

Terry weighed 116 pounds in her "before" picture, taken at thirty-eight years of age. Now, at forty-four, after one year of training, she weighs 114 pounds.

Terry is the mother of three children ranging from fifteen to nineteen years of age. She is a visual merchandiser for a major department store and is completing a degree in physical therapy. Terry tried aerobic programs, circuit training, dancing, tennis, and other gym programs. "I joined a popular health spa, and all they gave me were some light weights and told me to do ten reps and move to another machine. I kept at it for a year, but nothing happened. After all my efforts, I still had loads of cellulite, and my upper body was much smaller than my lower body. That's why now I've decided to devote some time to helping other women who mean business to train efficiently, so they can see results and not waste their time."

Terry says about starting, "I loved it and hated it at the same time. It all felt so foreign. Even holding the weights was odd. But after about a month I began to see some cellulite melt away, and I noticed my arms and shoulders beginning to change. It took about six months to really see results in my stomach and legs, and even a little longer for my back and other parts, but in time it all came together."

As for finding the time, Terry says, "I believe that women who say they can't find the time really don't want to do it. I work a nine-to-five job, have a husband and three children, and have lots of other responsibilities, yet because I want the results I find the time."

Working out has given Terry a new freedom. "I'm free from the scale now. I never bother to weigh myself. Who cares if I weigh 100 or 120. It's what I see in the mirror that counts, and I know others see it, too. I get more attention from men than I really want, but I like that problem. I never had it before."

I asked Terry what she feels is the best thing about this program. Unhesitatingly she replied, "The results."

BEFORE AND AFTER **221**

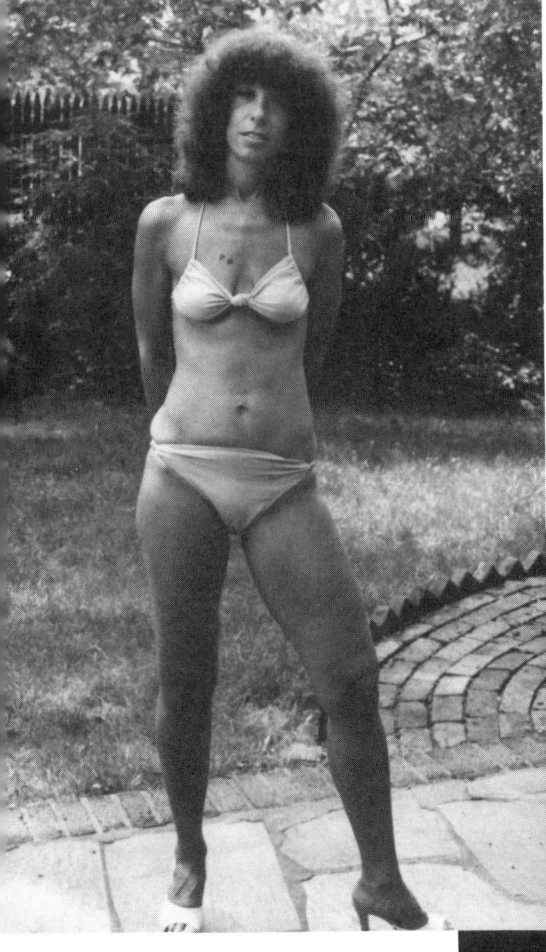

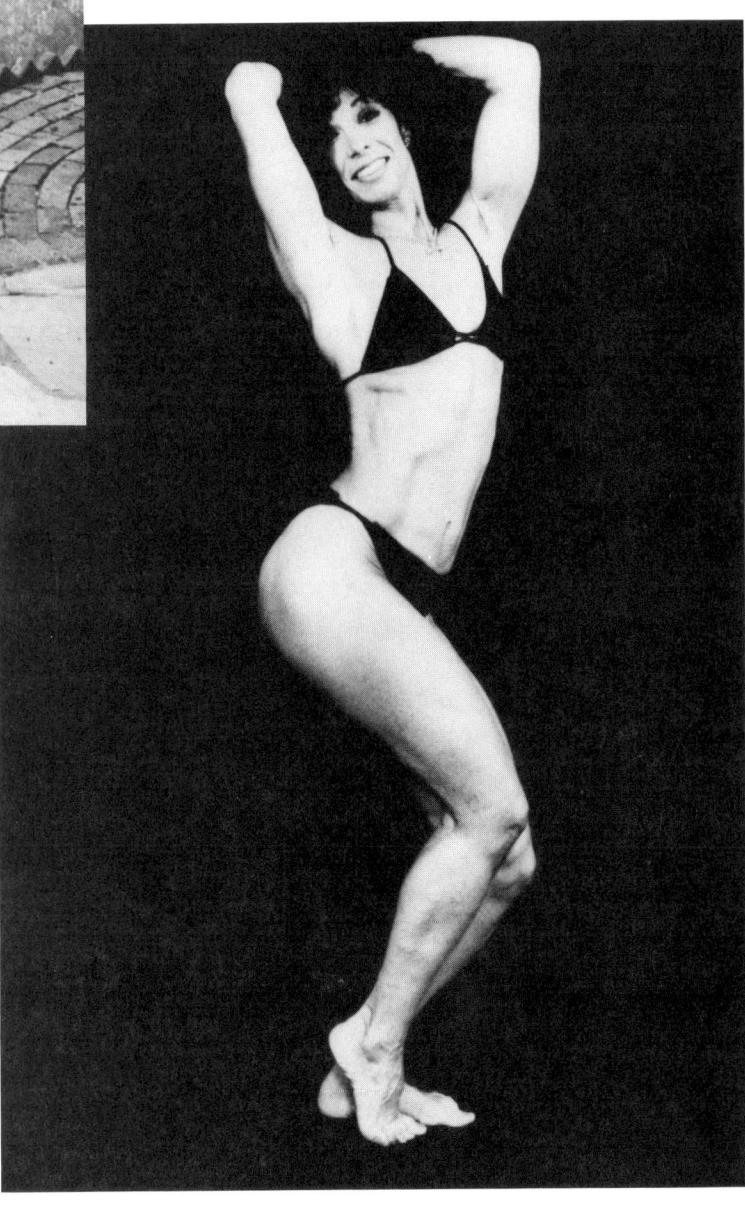

Before (116 pounds)

After one year
(114 pounds)

ELLEN CARTER, 33

Ellen is thirty-three years old in her "before" picture and she weighs 147 pounds. She is four months older in her "after" picture and weighs 127 pounds. She is still working on becoming the "perfect" body. In another eight months she ought to see even more progress.

Ellen is the mother of a ten-year-old son. She is a financial aid counselor and a professional musician. Ellen tried many fitness programs—"All sorts of diets—Pritikin, high-protein, quick weight-loss diet—the pulley system of exercise, and nothing worked. I would go up and down the scale like a yo-yo, and my body was still out of shape no matter what."

Ellen started working out with weights not really believing that it would work for her. "I always thought I was a special case. 'It may work for everyone else, but not me,' I thought. But after the first couple of weeks, when I noticed that my entire body seemed to be getting tighter even though the scale didn't show any difference, I became encouraged. I kept at it, and it did get better and better. Soon I began to lose weight."

When I asked Ellen why she didn't quit even though she was all aches and pains the next day, she said, "I could hardly get up the morning after the first workout, but I told myself I'd rather go through this pain than look the way I looked. [Ellen insisted upon doing all three sets per exercise on her first workout.] Anyway, I didn't want to be a quitter. Then, after two and a half months, I was to the point where if you told me I couldn't go to the gym I would say, 'No. I'm going. We'll have to work the other stuff around it.'"

Ellen has to work around it quite a bit. Here's her schedule: "I get up at five forty-five to check and help my son with his homework. He's having trouble this year. Then we eat breakfast, and I drive him to school. I go to work until five, and then I go to the gym (four days a week). After that I go home, make dinner, do household activities, and work on my music awhile. Two nights a week I go to the university, where I'm working on a second master's. I make the time to work out because I love the way I'm looking. It's worth it."

I asked Ellen if she thought other women could handle this program. "I was a total bookworm. I was the last person in the world who could ever be talked into doing something like this, and I was stubborn, thinking of reasons why it couldn't—wouldn't—work. But after a few weeks I started seeing the results, and now I believe that if I could do it—really, I'm not kidding—anyone can do it. I was and still am totally nonathletic."

I asked Ellen what the best part of working out is, and this is her reply: "Although I love the physical results, I have to say that for me the very best part is the effect it has on my mind. It helps me to see that no matter what things look like on the surface, one shouldn't look just at the circumstances. If you believe, you're going to be able to get through *anything*."

BEFORE AND AFTER

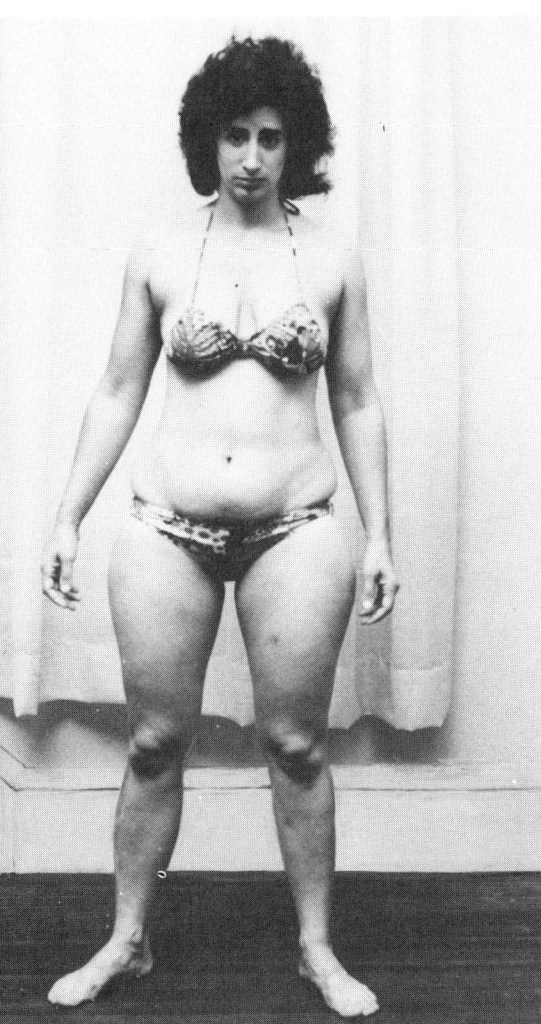

Before (147 pounds)

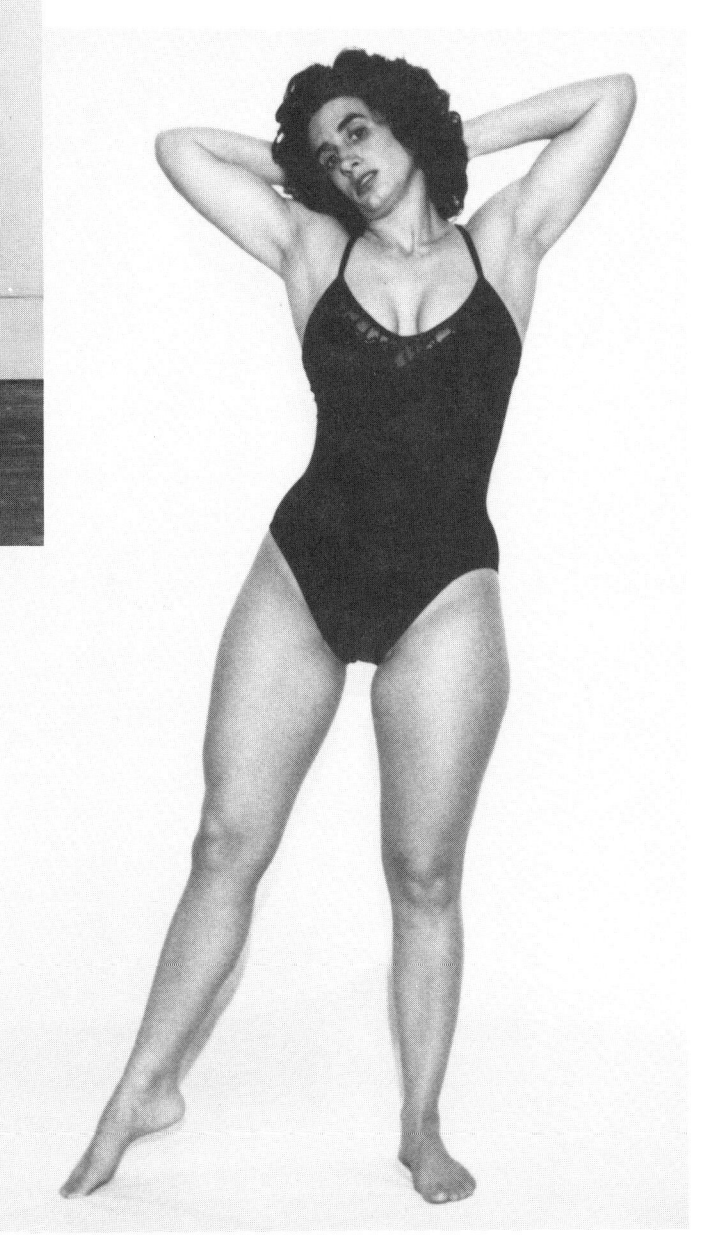

After four months
(127 pounds)

BARBARA VALE, 43

Barbara is forty-three years old in her "before" picture and weighs 155 pounds. In her second picture, she is three months older, and weighs 14 pounds less (141). In the third picture, she is yet another three months older (six months into the program) and weighs 128 pounds. She's still not at her goal—Barbara has another six months to go before she reaches her "perfect" body shape—but she's well on her way.

Barbara is the mother of three children ranging in age from five to seventeen. After working as an executive secretary, Barbara retired from that position to devote herself to helping her husband run his retail and real estate businesses. She now spends some of her time helping other women get into shape.

Barbara tried many programs before discovering this one. "I tried Weight Watchers five different times. I would lose a few pounds and gain them right back. I tried Elaine Powers twice, five years ago and two years ago. Both times I quit after a few months because I saw no results. None of those programs gave me an incentive to watch my diet. With this program, because I saw results in three weeks, I got psyched. I would sweat so hard and work so hard that I didn't want to blow it all by eating. And besides, the diet in this program is so reasonable. I am eating 1800 calories. I'm losing slowly, but I'm enjoying life, and I know the weight loss is permanent."

When I asked Barbara how she felt getting started, she laughed. "The gym owner was really negative. He didn't even want me to pay the full year. He said, 'Look, lady, I'll take your money, but if you want my advice you should pay for three months. I don't think you're going to stick with it.' (It was one of those mainly male bodybuilding gyms, but it was located right near my home, and I had the program so I didn't care what he said.) Despite what he said, I stuck with it, and now he's not only bragging about me, he's sending women over to me so I can help them."

Barbara suffered with a difficult body part, but other things encouraged her. "My legs were horrible. I remember that on the first day I thought I was going to do fifteen reps on the leg extension machine. All I could do was four reps. I was dying. The big thing was leaving the gym and walking down the stairs. I thought my legs would cave in under me. I remember having to think about each step. But the funny thing is, six weeks later I was thrilled to see my front thigh muscle developing. I guess it's because my legs were the weakest part to begin with."

I asked Barbara why she didn't quit the first few weeks. "I was desperate. I'd been gaining six to seven pounds a year for the past seven years. The first day was depressing and confusing. I had to look for every machine. But after I was totally committed—about three weeks—I noticed a biceps. I thought, It's now or never. Then every few weeks I would notice another part improving. In three months my behind changed; even my husband noticed it. Then my

BEFORE AND AFTER 225

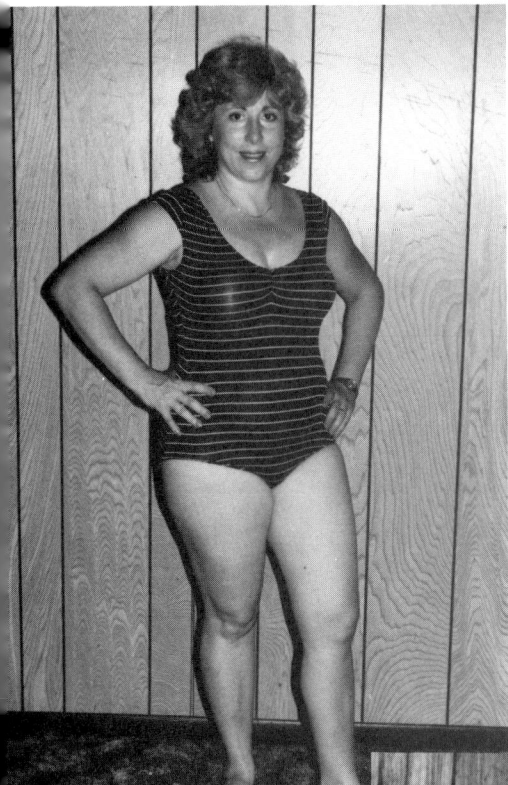

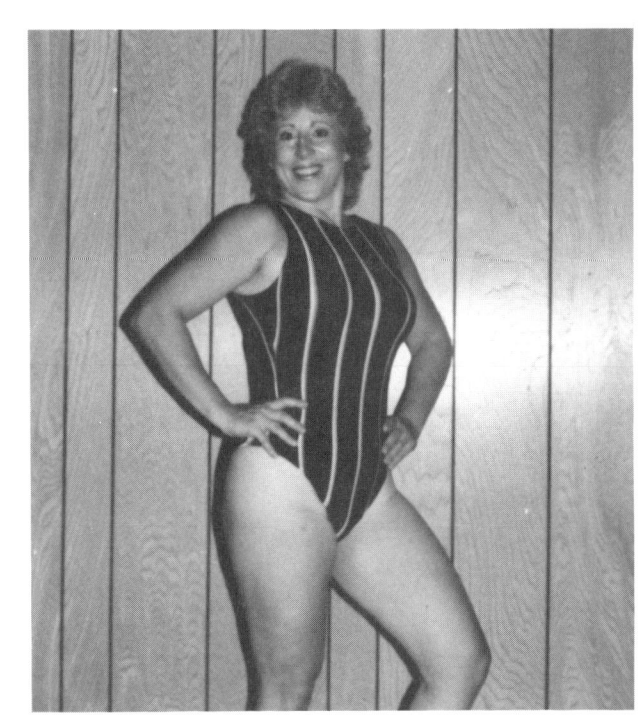

Before (155 pounds)

After three months (141 pounds)

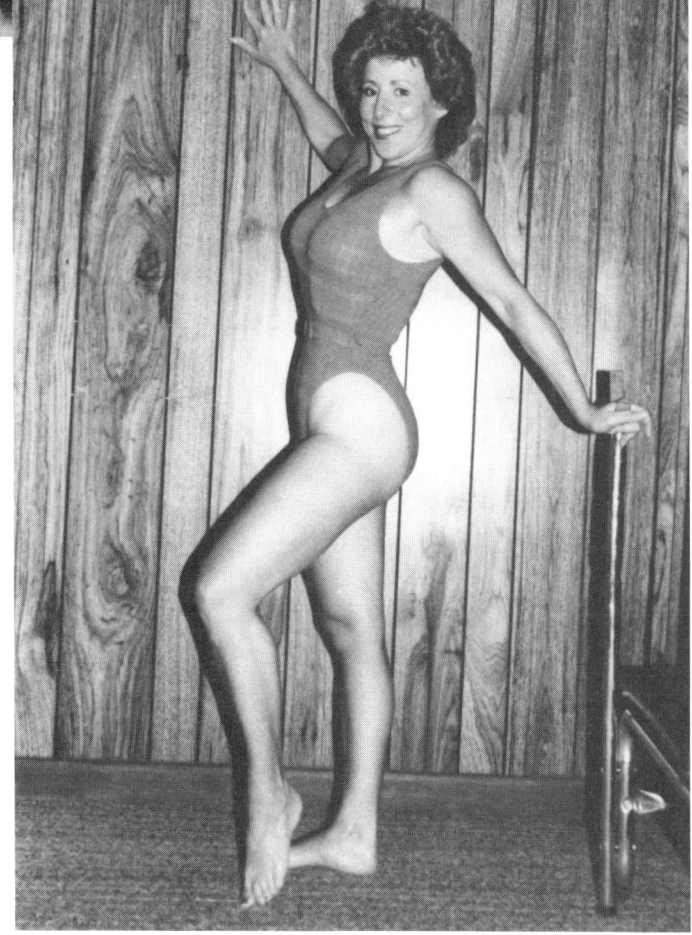

After six months (128 pounds)

stomach. I saw lines forming in my upper abdominal area, even though I still had lots of fat to lose. I thought, No way will I quit. It took me a long time to get this out of shape, and it may take a while to get into shape, but this works. I would never give it up.

"The thing is, I'm not only losing fat, I'm putting muscle there. My skin won't sag. It's adhering to good muscle. My husband likes it, too. He's always complimenting me, and for the first time people are not just saying, 'Barbara, you're losing weight.' They're saying, 'You look great! Your whole body is changing.'"

I asked Barbara what the best thing about working out is for her.

"It changed my whole mental attitude. I hated my body. It's reversing that. Also it carries over in a lot of ways—even to doing the bookwork for the businesses. Now I tell myself, 'Get up and do it.' I have ways to drive myself. I love it."

WHAT IS SO SPECIAL ABOUT THESE WOMEN?

None of these women have time to waste. They are very busy, just as you are, yet they devote the time because they like the results.

Every one of these women hated the way her body looked in the nude. "Disgusting. I wouldn't look. I was ashamed. Horrible." These are the words they use to describe the way they felt about their "before" bodies.

Each woman had to overcome the temptation to give in to initial insecurity, confusion, and pain, to surrender to the urge to quit. And yet each of them, out of desperation from having tried everything else, forged ahead and was hooked within three weeks to a month.

Though the women in this chapter come from different backgrounds, they shared a common desire to get in shape. But there was something more they shared. They had a goal, and they were determined to achieve it. They had made up their minds that nothing was going to stop them. No matter what, they would tough it out.

I notice a similar determination in other women I introduce to this program. The ones who succeed are always the ones who mean business.

After two weeks of training, Sandy, a forty-one-year-old bookstore owner, was so excited about her workout that it was almost impossible to get her to rest more than ten seconds between sets. In addition she insisted upon doing all three sets by the end of the second week. "I was meant for this," she says. "It was a long time coming, but now that I've started, I'm not fooling around here. Let's get on with it."

If women like Sandy, Barbara, Ellen, Terry, and Roberta can do it, so can you. Make the decision to start today. Place your "before" picture in the space provided. Then every three months take an "after" to record your progress. You'll be amazed. You'll be delighted.

What's it going to be? A body that's a few pounds heavier or unsatisfyingly the same a year from now or the totally transformed body of a determined woman who said, *"Now or never,"* and then took action?

Place your own before and after pictures here.

Before   After

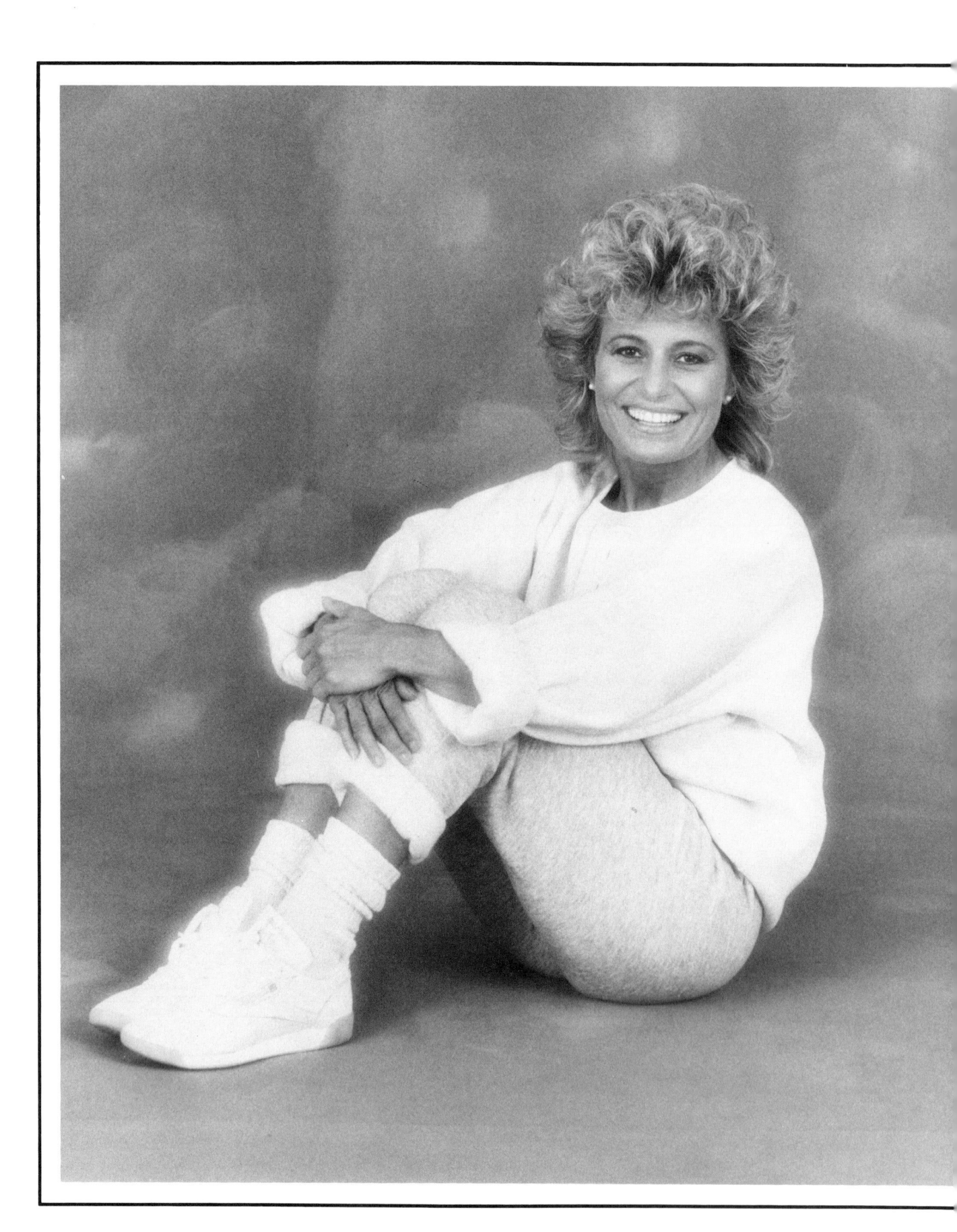

CHAPTER 12

FOREVER FIT

This program comes with a lifetime guarantee of fitness... if you keep it up. Fortunately, there is little danger of your wanting to stop working out once you become "addicted." This process takes anywhere from one day to three months.

You may be like Carla, a forty-three-year-old housewife who, when asked how long it took her to become addicted, immediately answered, "One day. I loved it. There was no way I would ever quit after my first workout. I remember how surprised the gym owner was to see me back the next day. He said, 'Back again? After all that work you did yesterday I thought you'd quit.'" He had tried to convince Carla that this workout would be too much for her. She simply ignored him and did everything prescribed in the workout.

There are some other things to consider, however. What happens in the event of a life crisis, when it is necessary to miss a few workouts, or in the case of a vacation or an injury? Nothing. You simply miss a workout or two—or ten or a hundred—but you get right back on track as soon as that is humanly possible.

Vacations are actually good for your workout. I spent four weeks in Italy, drinking wine and eating delicious Italian food. I then returned to my workout, and five weeks later was in the best shape of my life. I entered a major bodybuilding contest and placed high.

When your body is used to working out and then is forced to rest, it remains in a state of readiness, longing for the missed stimulation. The moment the muscles are again stimulated they virtually jump back into shape, and with that jump they make additional gains. A forced rest can be a blessing in disguise.

Even when your workout recess is longer than desired, keep in mind that it takes less than one-third as long as the initial building period to restore lost muscles.

YOU'LL NEVER QUIT!

I asked hundreds of women who had been working out for more than three months (the time range was from three months to five years) how they would respond if someone told them they could never work out again. Each woman became emotional about it. Each stated emphatically that she would never, under any conditions, give this up. They all agreed that working out had changed their entire outlook on life. It gave them a new feeling about their bodies and a concurrent sense of self-confidence and power. In addition, each women reports that she is no longer ashamed of her body in the nude. They all affirm that they would find some way to work around any obstacle that might come in the way of working out. Under no circumstances would they give up their workout program.

Did You Give It Your Best Shot?

The only reason you might quit is that you are having a difficult time making it through the initial break-in period. That is when you will be wondering, "Can I do it? Will this work for *me*?"

You owe it to yourself to fight your way through those early difficult days. If you gave up, could you honestly say, "I couldn't have done any better if someone had held a gun to my head"? That's what I always ask myself when I seem to be failing at a new task. Did I really give it all I had? And if the answer is no, I go back twice as determined as before to overcome the obstacle.

Take a chance. Try it. Give it your best shot. Don't give in to weakness, fear, or negative thinking. Don't let the chorus of skeptical commentators get you down. Show them! Soon they'll be coming to you for advice.

Soon You'll Be on Automatic

It won't be long before working out becomes as natural to you as taking a daily shower or fixing breakfast. Less and less conscious effort need be invested as you learn to go "on automatic." You will take the efforts you make for granted and wonder why people think it is so remarkable that you devote six hours a week to your fitness program. It will seem as necessary and natural to work out as it is to do the food shopping or brush your teeth. You won't really miss the time it takes, because you will have learned to cut corners, shearing time off telephone conversations, television viewing, and other expendable activities.

LOOK AT YOU!

Proud in the nude. Finally. That's how you will feel in a year's time.

One of the worst things for a woman is to think of her out-of-shape body when it is about to be exposed to someone who thinks she looks great in clothing. No longer will you dread this awful moment of truth.

Proud on the beach. Finally. That's how you will feel in a year's time.

One of the most depressing thoughts a woman can experience is "How will I hide my flabby body at the beach." No longer will you have to think about concealing yourself.

Proud in the gym. Finally. That's how you will feel in a year's time. You will know that you belong, that you are a fitness expert and that bodybuilding is your sport. No longer will you feel out of place and awkward around other people when exercising your body.

Proud in your walk. Finally. That's how you will feel in a year's time. Your stride will be confident and athletic. Your firm arms will swing freely, complemented by shapely shoulder muscles and *V*-shaped lats. No longer will you shuffle along with poor posture. You will never have to walk that way again.

Proud in your mind. Finally. That's how you will feel in a year's time. No longer will you tell yourself, "I can't." You will know that you can, that you did, that you will. Your success in conquering your body will carry over into other areas of life. You will never readily accept defeat again.

Finally!

Bibliography

Becker, Robert O., M.D., and Gary Seldon. *The Body Electric: Electromagnetism and the Foundation of Life.* New York: William Morrow and Company, 1985.
Blakeslee, Thomas R. *The Right Brain: A New Understanding of the Unconscious Mind and Its Creative Powers.* New York: Playboy Paperbacks, 1980.
Boswell, Nelson. *Successful Living Day by Day.* New York: The Macmillan Company, 1972.
Bristol, Claude M. *The Magic of Believing.* New York: Pocket Books, 1948.
Cousins, Norman. *The Healing Heart.* New York: Avon Books, 1983.
Dardik, Irving, M.D., F.A.C.S., and Dennis Waitley, Ph.D. *Quantum Fitness.* New York: Simon and Schuster, 1984.
Dyer, Wayne. *Pulling Your Own Strings.* New York: Avon Books, 1977.
Feinberg, Gerald. *Solid Clues. Quantum Physics, Molecular Biology and the Future of Science.* New York: Simon and Schuster, 1985.
Friedberg, Ardy. *Reach for It.* New York: Simon and Schuster, 1983.
Haas, Robert, Ph.D. *Eat to Win—The Sports Nutrition Bible.* New York: Rawson Associates, 1983.
Hausman, Patricia. *At-a-Glance Nutrition Counter.* New York: Ballantine Books, 1984.
Jacobson, Michael, M.D., and Bonnie F. Liebman and Greg Moyer. *Salt: The Brand Name Guide to Sodium Content.* New York: Workman Publishing Company, 1983.
Jerome, John. *Staying with It.* New York: The Viking Press, 1984.
Kirschmann, John, Editor. *The Nutrition Almanac.* New York: McGraw-Hill Book Company, 1979.

Krieger, Dolores, Ph.D., R.N. *The Therapeutic Touch.* Englewood Cliffs, New Jersey: Prentice-Hall, 1979.

Maltz, Maxwell, M.D., F.I.C.S. *The Magic Power of Self-Image Psychology.* Englewood Cliffs, New Jersey: Prentice-Hall, 1964.

———. *Psychocybernetics.* Englewood Cliffs, New Jersey: Prentice-Hall, 1960.

Ornstein, Robert. *The Psychology of Consciousness.* New York: Harcourt Brace Jovanovich, 1977.

Peale, Norman Vincent. *The Positive Principle Today.* Englewood Cliffs, New Jersey: Prentice-Hall, 1976.

———. *You Can If You Think You Can.* Englewood Cliffs, New Jersey: Prentice-Hall, 1975.

Reynolds, Bill, and Joyce Vedral, Ph.D. *Supercut: Nutrition for the Ultimate Physique.* Chicago: Contemporary Books, 1985.

Schuller, Robert H. *You Can Become the Person You Want to Be.* New York: Hawthorn Books, 1973.

Vaughan, William, M.D. *Low Sugar Secrets for Your Diet.* New York: Warner Books, 1985.

Weinberg, George. *The Pliant Animal.* New York: St. Martin's Press, 1981.

Williams, John K. *The Knack of Using Your Subconscious Mind: How to Tap Your Inner Power.* Englewood Cliffs, New Jersey: Prentice-Hall, 1980.

Wilson, Donald, M.D. *Total Mind Power.* New York: Berkley Books, 1978.

Wood, Paul E., M.D. *How to Get Yourself to Do What You Want to Do.* Englewood Cliffs, New Jersey: Prentice-Hall, 1981.

MAGAZINES

Muscle and Beauty, 888 Seventh Avenue, New York, NY 10106.

Muscle and Fitness, 21100 Erwin Street, Woodland Hills, CA 91367.

Shape, 21100 Erwin Street, Woodland Hills, CA 91367.

Strength Training for Beauty, 1400 Stierlin Road, Mountain View, CA 94043.

About the Author

Joyce Vedral, Ph.D., is an assistant professor of English at Pace University in New York City. She is the author of *Hard Bodies*, with Gladys Portugues, a fitness book for women, and *Supercut*, with Bill Reynolds, a book on diet and nutrition. She has also written two advice books for teenagers: *I Dare You* and *My Parents Are Driving Me Crazy*.

Joyce is a regular contributor to *Muscle and Fitness* magazine, and has been featured on the cover of *Muscle and Beauty* magazine. She has been interviewing and training with champion bodybuilders for the past five years. She has participated in many sports, among them mountain climbing, the martial arts, running, and tennis. Joyce has discovered that the only way to reshape the body into perfect form is to work out with weights—*the right way.*

This author has a thirteen-year-old daughter, holds a full-time job, writes books and magazine articles and yet maintains her physical condition. She follows the workout described in this book. Try it.

Index

—A—

Abdominal routine, 138–45
  bench leg raise, 142–43
  crunch, 140–41
  leg-in, 144–45
  sit-ups, straight and incline, 138–39
Abdominals, 50, 72, 138–45
  defined, 50
  pyramiding and, 72
  routine for, 138–45
Aerobic fitness, 3, 7, 40–42, 79–80, 200
  beginning sessions, 79–80
  choices of exercises, 41
  fallacy about, 7
  optimum heart-lung stimulation, 40
  removing excess fat and, 40
  scheduling sessions, 40–42
  stationary bicycle and, 41
  swimming and, 41
  three 20-minute sessions, 40
  walking and, 41
  weeks one through four, 79–80
  weight-loss diet and, 200
Aging, 2, 3–4, 5, 9n, 12–13, 31–32, 190
  activity and, 12–13
  confused with being out of shape, 12
  cosmetic surgery and, 3–4
  defined, 9n
  middle years and, 2
  mind control and, 31–32
  skin and, 5
  weight-gain myth and, 190
Alcohol, 29, 207
  calories and, 207
  energy level and, 207
Anabolic steroids, 6

—B—

Back, defined, 50
Back leg kick, 150–51
Back routines, 104–11
  lat machine pulldown to back, 104–05
  lat machine pulldown to front, 110–11
  one-arm dumbbell bent row, 108–09
  seated pulley row, 106–07
Balanced diet, 194–95
Barbells, 53
Barbell tuck, 152–53
Basic equipment. *See* Equipment

Becker, Dr. Robert O., 59–60, 65n
Before-and-after profiles, 217–227
"Before" photos, 218
Beginner's routines, 8
Beland, Irene, 209n
Bench leg raise, 142–43
Bench press, 88–89
Bent-knee deadlifts, 166–67
Biceps, defined, 50
Biceps routine, 112–19
    concentration curl, 114–15
    incline dumbbell curl, 118–119
    one-arm preacher curl, 114–15
    standing barbell curl, 112–13
Blood sugar levels, 191
Body condition, 11–19
    activity and, 12–13
    addictiveness of training, 18–19
    aging and, 12
    body types and, 14–15
    losing muscle, 18
    mirror image and, 17
    neglected muscles, 13
    overweight and, 14
    stopping workouts, 17–18
    too light in weight, 14
    triceps muscle and, 13
Body Electric, The (Becker and Seldon), 59–60, 65n
Body parts, 47–51
    abdominals, 50
    back, 50
    biceps, 50
    buttocks, 50
    chest, 50
    legs, 51
    shoulders, 50
    triceps, 50
Body types, 14–15
    ectomorphs, 14–15
    endomorphs, 14–15
    mesomorphs, 14–15
Body weight, 14–17
    body types and, 14–15
    mirrors and, 17
    muscle *vs.* fat, 15–17
Bombing, 211–15
    additional sets, 214–15
    burns and, 214
    cheating and, 213
    common troublesome areas, 215
    extra days and, 215
    forced reps and, 213
    muscle priority training and, 212
    spot reducing, 211–12
    "training to failure" and, 213-14
    when to use, 212
Boswell, Nelson, 35n
Breathing, 85–86
Burns, 214
Buttocks, 50, 72, 146–53
    defined, 50
    pyramiding, 72
    routine, 146–53
Buttocks routine, 146–53
    back leg kick, 150–51
    barbell tuck, 152–53
    feather kick-up, 146–47
    scissors, 148–49

—C—

Cable crossover, 94–95
Calories, 189
Carbohydrates, 189, 191–92, 195, 198–99, 203
    complex, 192
    excessive intake of, 192
    processed, 191
    simple, 192
    weight-gain diet and, 203
    weight-loss diet and, 198–99
Carter, Ellen, 222–23
Cheating, 213
Chest, 50, 88–95
    defined, 50
    routine, 88–95
Chest routine, 88–95
    bench press, 88–89
    cable crossover, 94–95
    cross bench pullover, 92–93
    incline flye, 90–91
Cholesterol, 194
Circuit training, 5, 13, 82
Clinical Nursing: Pathophysiological and Psychosocial Approaches (Beland and Passos), 209n
Clothing for workouts, 78–79
Collars, 54
Common areas of trouble, 215
Complex carbohydrates, 192
Concentration, 31, 60–61
    defined, 60
    "working in" and, 61
Concentration curl, 116–17
Condition. *See* Body condition
Cosmetic surgery, 3–4
Cousins, Norman, 58–59, 65n
Cross bench pullover, 92–93
Crunch, 140–41

—D—

Dardik, Irving, 35n
Decline bench press, 158–59
Definition, 54
Density, 54
Diet, 7, 28–29, 186–209
    alcohol and, 207
    balanced diet, 194–95
    blood sugar levels and, 191
    calories and, 189
    carbohydrates and, 189, 191–192, 195
    eating before workouts, 207
    fad diets, 206
    fats, 194, 195
    "forbidden foods," 188, 204–05
    habit and, 188
    maintenance diet, 204–06
    mind control and, 28–29
    MSG and, 188, 196
    points to remember about, 208
    protein, 193, 195
    sodium and, 188, 195–97
    as "usual food and drink," 187–88
    visualization and, 28–29
    water, 197
    weight-gain diet, 202–04
    weight-loss diet, 198–200
    weight loss, 189–90
Dieting, 7, 206
    fad diets, 206
    See also Weight-gain diet; Weight-loss diet; Weight loss
Dips between benches, 126–27
Dumbbell kickback, 174–75
Dumbbell leg curl, 180–81
Dumbbells, defined, 54
Dyer, Dr. Wayne, 35n

INDEX

E

Eat to Win: The Sports Nutrition Bible (Hass), 209n
Ectomorphs, 14–15
Endomorphs, 14–15
Equipment, 53–54, 83
   barbells, 53
   collars, 54
   dumbbells, 54
   flat exercise bench, 53
   free weights, 54
   for home workouts, 83
   incline exercise bench, 53
   machines, 54
"Exercise," defined, 51

F

Fad diets, 206
Fascia injuries, 56
Fat (body fat), 189–90
   age and, 190
   ideal amount, 190
   muscle *vs.,* 189
   women and, 190
Fat (in diet), 194, 195, 199
   cholesterol and, 194
   excessive intake of, 194, 195
   function of, 194
   weight-loss diet and, 199
Feather kick-up, 146–47
Feinberg, Dr. Gerald, 9n
First week, 68–70
   first day, 68–69
   second day, 69–70
   third and fourth days, 70
Fitness fallacies, 7
Flat exercise bench, 53
Flex, 45n, 83
Flexing, defined, 31
"Forbidden foods," 188, 204–205
Forced repetitions, 213
Forty pounds overweight, 45
Four-session split routines, 38–39
Free weights, 54
Friedberg, Ardy, 83n
Front lateral raise, 98–99

G

Gym workouts, 80–82, 85–153
   abdominal routine, 138–45
   back routine, 104–11
   beginning weight, 86
   biceps routine, 112–19
   breathing, 85–86
   buttocks routine, 146–53
   chest routine, 88–96
   choosing a gym, 81–82
   circuit training and, 82
   health spas and, 81–82
   home workouts *vs.,* 80–81
   leg routine, 128–37
   order of exercises, 86
   overview of, 85
   pros and cons of, 81
   shoulder routine, 96–103
   triceps routine, 120–27

H

Haas, Dr. Robert, 195, 209n
Healing, 57–60
Healing Heart, The (Cousins), 58–59
Health spas, 81–82
Home workouts, 80–81, 83, 155–85
   about abdominal routine, 182
   bent-knee deadlifts, 166–67
   about buttocks routine, 184
   decline bench press, 158–159
   dumbbell kickback, 174–75
   dumbbell leg curl, 180–81
   equipment for, 83
   gym workouts *vs.,* 80–81
   seated dumbbell rear laterals, 164–65
   spinal lifts, 162–63
   standing alternating dumbbell curl, 170–71
   standing leg extension, 178–79
   See also Abdominal routine; Back routine; Biceps routine; Buttocks routine; Chest routine; Leg routine; Shoulder routine
How to Get Yourself to Do What You Want to Do (Wood), 29, 35n, 201n

I

Incline dumbbell curl, 118–19
Incline exercise bench, 53
Incline flye, 90–91
Injury(ies), 19, 55–58
   accepting, 57
   "claiming it" and, 58
   electrical stimulation for, 60
   evaluating seriousness of, 57
   fascia, 56
   induced healing of, 57–60
   ligament, 56
   tendonitus, 56
   warmup exercises and, 56
   working around, 56–57

J

Jerome, John, 12

K

Krieger, Dolores, 59, 65n

L

Lat machine pulldown to back, 104–05
Lat machine pulldown to front, 110–11
Left brain, 26–27
   as "input," 27
   -right brain combination, 27
Leg-in, 144–45
Leg curl, 134–35
Leg extension, 132–33, 178–79
   standing, 178–79
Leg routine, 128–37
   leg curl, 134–35
   leg extension, 132–33
   lunge, 128–29
   one-leg toe raise, 136–37
   squat, 130–31
Legs, defined, 51
Lemon juice, 201
Ligament injuries, 56
Lombardi, Vince, 24

Lunge, 128–29
Lying triceps extension, 122–23

M

Machines, 54
Maintaining training, 229–32
    as automatic, 231
    "best shot" and, 230–31
    "lifetime guarantee" and, 229
    pride and, 231–32
    quitting, 230
Maintenance diet, 204–06
    calories allowed, 204
    "forbidden foods" and, 204–205
    general guidelines for, 204
    metabolism and, 204
    muscular women and, 204
    physical activity and, 204
    setting weight limits, 205
    weight-gain and, 205
Maltz, Maxwell, 27, 35n
Martial arts, 13
McLish, Rachel, 38
Mesomorphs, 14–15
Metabolism, 29–31, 202, 204
    mind control and, 29–31
    weight-loss diet and, 202
Military press behind neck, 100–101
Mind control, 21–35
    aging and, 31–32
    body influenced by, 23–25
    careers and, 23
    diet changes and, 28–29
    gradual change and, 22
    inner balance and, 21
    left brain and, 26–27
    listening to the body, 24–25
    maturity and, 22
    metabolism speedup and, 29–31
    motivation and, 25
    muscle buildup and, 31
    negative attitudes, 24, 32–33
    personality and, 22–23
    positive thinking and, 32–33
    right brain and, 26
    spot picturing, 29
    "under twenty" and, 34
    visualization and, 27–28
Mirrors, as measuring devices, 17

Motivation, 25
Muscle(s):
    consciousness, 76–78
    definition, 54
    density, 54
    fat and, 15, 189–90
    injury and, 55–58
    investment in, 18
    isolation, 4
    mind control and, 31
    pump, defined, 54
    soreness of, 55
    stopping workouts and, 17–18
Muscle and Fitness, 5, 45n, 83
Muscle consciousness, 76–78
    flexing, 77
    soreness and, 77–78
    stretching, 77
    visualization and, 77
Muscle priority training, 212
Muscularity, 6
    professional bodybuilders, 6
    steroids and, 6
    testosterone and, 6
MSG, 188, 196

N

Nautilus machines, 54
Negative attitudes, 24, 32–33
    positive attitudes *vs.,* 32–33
    restating negative thoughts, 33
    verbalizing negative thoughts, 33
Nutrition Almanac, The, 191, 199

O

One-arm dumbbell bent row, 108–09
One-arm dumbbell triceps extension, 120–21
One-arm preacher curl, 114–15
One-leg toe raise, 136–37
Ornstein, Dr. Robert, 60, 65n
Out of shape, *See* Body condition
Overweight women, 14, 15

P

Paragon machines, 54
Partners. *See* Training partners; Spotters
Passos, Joyce Y., 209n
Perine, Terry, 220–21
"Phosphorus jitters," 193
Plates, 54
Positive thinking, 32–33
    negative thinking *vs.,* 32–33
    restating negative thoughts, 33
Problem areas. *See* Bombing
Processed carbohydrates, 191
Progression, 52
Protein, 193, 195, 199, 203
    complete, 193
    incomplete, 193
    "phosphorus jitters" and, 193
    weight-gain diet and, 203
    weight-loss diet and, 199
Psychocybernetics (Maltz), 35n
Psychology of Consciousness, The (Ornstein), 65n
Pulley pushdown, 124–25
Pulling Your Own Strings (Dyer), 35n
Pump, defined, 42, 54
Pyramiding, 3, 52–53, 71–72, 72–73
    abdominals and, 72
    buttocks and, 72
    defined, 52–53
    in second week, 71–72
    in third week, 72–73
    weights and, 75

Q

Quantum Fitness (Dardik and Waitley), 35n

R

Reach for It (Friedberg), 83n
Repetitions (reps), 51, 213
    forced, 213

Rest, defined, 51–52
Results of weight training, 42–45
   one month, 43
   one year, 44
   overweight and, 45
   six months, 44
   three months, 43
   three weeks, 42
   two months, 43
Reynolds, Bill, 196
Right brain, 26–27
Robinson, Roberta, 218–19
Routine, defined, 52
Running, 13

S

Skin care, 5
   circulatory stimulation, 5
   water and, 5
Salt, 196
   See also Sodium
Scheduling, 39–40
   choosing beginning day, 39
   regular routines, 40
   times of day, 39
   weekends and, 39
Schuller, Robert H., 19n, 33
Schwarzenegger, Arnold, 38
Scissors, 148–49
Seated dumbbell rear laterals, 164–65
Seated pulley row, 106–07
Second week, 71–72
   pyramiding, 71–72
Seldon, Gary, 65n
Sets, defined, 51
Shape, 45n
Shoulder routine, 96–103
   front lateral raise, 98–99
   military press behind neck, 100–01
   side lateral raise, 96–97
   upright row, 102–03
Shoulders, defined, 50
Side lateral raise, 96–97
Simple carbohydrates, 192
Sit-ups, straight and incline, 138–39
Sodium, 188, 195–97
   "allowance" for, 196
   function of, 195
   recommended intake of, 196
   table salt, 196
   water retention and, 196

Soreness, 55, 77–78
   causes of, 55
   delight with, 55
   exception of, 77–78
   working through, 55
Spinal lifts, 162–63
Split routines, 3, 38, 53
   defined and described, 53
Sports Fitness, 45n
Spot picturing, 29
Spot reducing, *See* Bombing
Spotters, 65
   See also Training partners
Squat, 130–31
Standing alternating dumbbell curl, 170–71
Standing barbell curl, 112–13
Standing leg extension, 178–179
Stationary bicycle, 41
Staying with It (Jerome), 12
Steroids, 6
Stopping workouts, 17–18
   losing muscle, 18
   muscle and fat, 17–18
Successful Living Day by Day (Boswell), 35n
Supercut (Reynolds and Vedral), 196
Swimming, 41

T

Tendonitus, 56
Testosterone, 6
Therapeutic Touch, The (Krieger), 59, 65n
Third week, 72–73
   full pyramiding and, 72–73
Timing, 37–45
   four sessions a week, 38–39
   one-day-a-week workouts, 38
   results at various stages, 42–44
   scheduling, 39–40
   split routines and, 38
   streamlined program and, 37
   three-day-a-week workouts, 38
   twice-a-week workouts, 38
Total body lift, 1–9
   aerobic fitness and, 3, 7
   aging process and, 2
   cosmetic surgery and, 3–4

   dieting and, 7
   fallacies about fitness, 7
   skin care, 5
Total Mind Power (Wilson), 28, 35n, 209n
Training partners, 64–65
   incentive and, 64
   last rep and, 64–65
   spotters, 65
   slowing down with, 64
"Training to failure," 213–14
   burns 214
   cheating, 213
   forced repetitions, 213
   how to use, 214
Triceps, 13, 50
Triceps routine, 120–27
   dips between benches, 126–127
   lying triceps extension, 122–123
   one-arm dumbbell triceps extension, 120–21

U

Universal Gym machines, 54
Upright row, 102–03

V

Vale, Barbara, 224–25
Vedral, Joyce, 196
Vinegar, 201
Visualization, 27–28, 29, 62–63, 77, 201
   diet and, 28–29
   in the gym, 63
   mirrors and, 28, 62–63
   negative images and, 63
   spot picturing, 29
   weight-loss diet and, 201

W

Waitley, Dennis, 27, 35n
Walking, 41
Warmup exercises, 56, 67–68
   injuries and, 56

INDEX

Water, 196, 197
  amounts to drink, 197
  importance to body, 197
  sodium and, 196, 197
  system flushed by, 197
Weight-gain diet, 202–03
  calorie-intake increase, 202–203
  carbohydrates and, 203
  protein and, 203
Weight-loss diet, 198–202
  aerobics and, 200
  carbohydrates and, 198–99
  fats and, 199
  500-calorie reduction, 198
  frequent small meals, 200–201
  lemon juice and, 201
  losing pounds gradually, 198
  metabolism and, 202
  protein and, 199
  snacks, 201
  vinegar and, 201
  visualization and, 201
  See also Weight loss
Weight loss, 189–90
  age and, 190
  fat and, 190
  muscle *vs.* fat, 189–90
  See also Weight-loss diet
Weights, 74–76, 86
  increasing, 75–76
  lightest as "too heavy," 74
  pyramiding, 75
  selecting, 74–76, 86
Weight training:
  addictiveness of, 18–19
  aerobic fitness and, 3, 7, 40–42, 79–80
  before-and-after profiles, 217–27
  "beginner's routine" as time waster, 8
  body condition and, 11–19
  body types and, 14–15
  body weight and, 14–17
  bombing, 211–15
  changes in routine, 8, 9
  circuit training, 5
  determination and, 226–27
  diet and, 186–209
  effectiveness of weights, 3
  expectations and, 8
  failures with weights, 5–6
  first week, 68–70
  four-session split routines, 38–39
  gym workouts, 80–82, 85–153
  home workouts, 80–81, 155–85
  injuries and, 19, 55–58
  maintaining training, 229–32
  mind control and, 21–35
  muscle isolation and, 4
  ordered use of weights, 3
  personality and, 22–23
  pyramiding, 3, 52–53
  results of, 42–45
  sequence of training, 5
  six hours a week, 3
  split routines, 3
  stopping workouts, 17–18
  timing, 37–45
  total body lift, 1–9
  workout fundamentals, 47–65
  workouts (generally), 47–65
  workout preparations, 67–83
Weider, Joe, 38, 45n, 213
Wilson, Dr. Donald, 28, 31, 35n, 209n
Wood, Dr. Paul E., 29, 35n, 201
"Working in," 61
Workout fundamentals, 47–65
  body parts and, 47–51
  concentration, 60–61
  equipment, 53–54
  "exercise" defined, 51
  injuries and, 55–58
  language, 51–54
  muscle development, 54
  principles of, 52
  procedures, 51–52
  repetitions (reps), 51
  rests, 51–52
  "routine" defined, 52
  sets, 51
  soreness and, 55
  spotters, 65
  training partners, 64–65
  visualization and, 62–63
  "workout" defined, 52
  See also Workouts (generally); Workout preparation
Workout preparation, 67–83
  aerobics and, 79–80
  clothing, 78–79
  first week, 68–70
  gym *vs.* home, 80–81
  increasing weight, 75–76
  muscle consciousness, 76–78
  second week, 71–72
  selecting weights, 74–76
  third week, 72–73
  warmup stretching, 67–68
Workout principles, 52–53
  progression, 52
  pyramiding, 52–53
  split routine, 53
Workouts (generally), 47–65, 67–83, 85–153, 155–85, 207
  aerobics and, 79–80
  defined, 52
  eating before workouts, 207
  fundamentals, 47–65
  gym workouts, 80–82, 85–153
  home workouts, 80–81, 83, 155–85
  preparation, 67–83
  stopping workouts, 17–18
  therapeutic effects of working out, 64
  See also Workout fundamentals

Y

You Can Become the Person You Want to Be (Schuller), 19n